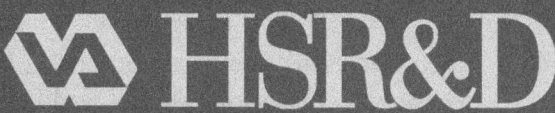

I0470652

A Systematic Evidence Review of the Signs and Symptoms of Dementia and Brief Cognitive Tests Available in VA

April 2010

Prepared for:

Department of Veterans Affairs

Veterans Health Administration

Health Services Research & Development Service

Washington, DC 20420

Prepared by:

VA Evidence-based Synthesis Program (ESP) Center

Portland VA Medical Center

Portland, OR

Devan Kansagara, MD, Director

Investigators:

Principal Investigator:

Devan Kansagara, MD

Research Associate:

Michele Freeman, MPH

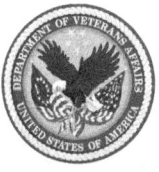

PREFACE

HSR&D's Evidence-based Synthesis Program (ESP) was established to provide timely and accurate syntheses of targeted healthcare topics of particular importance to VA managers and policymakers, as they work to improve the health and healthcare of Veterans. The ESP disseminates these reports throughout VA.

HSR&D provides funding for four ESP Centers and each Center has an active VA affiliation. The ESP Centers generate evidence syntheses on important clinical practice topics, and these reports help:

- develop clinical policies informed by evidence,

- the implementation of effective services to improve patient outcomes and to support VA clinical practice guidelines and performance measures, and

- set the direction for future research to address gaps in clinical knowledge.

In 2009, an ESP Coordinating Center was created to expand the capacity of HSR&D Central Office and the four ESP sites by developing and maintaining program processes. In addition, the Center established a Steering Committee comprised of HSR&D field-based investigators, VA Patient Care Services, Office of Quality and Performance, and VISN Clinical Management Officers. The Steering Committee provides program oversight and guides strategic planning, coordinates dissemination activities, and develops collaborations with VA leadership to identify new ESP topics of importance to Veterans and the VA healthcare system.

Comments on this evidence report are welcome and can be sent to Nicole Floyd, ESP Coordinating Center Program Manager, at nicole.floyd@va.gov.

Recommended citation: Kansagara D and Freeman M. A Systematic Evidence Review of the Signs and Symptoms of Dementia and Brief Cognitive Tests Available in VA. VA-ESP Project #05-225; 2010.

TABLE OF CONTENTS

EXECUTIVE SUMMARY

BACKGROUND

The Veterans Health Administration (VHA) Office of Geriatrics and Extended Care (OGEC) in Patient Care Services has primary responsibility for coordination and direction of VHA dementia initiatives. OGEC convened an interdisciplinary Dementia Steering Committee (DSC) in December 2006, with the goal of making recommendations on comprehensive, coordinated care for Veterans with dementia.

The DSC requested VA HSR&D's Evidence-based Synthesis Program (ESP) to review evidence on selected topics to assist with DSC planning efforts.

Broad-based dementia screening programs have not been widely advocated given lack of evidence that earlier detection will improve health outcomes. Improving the accuracy of case-finding techniques depends both on an understanding of signs and symptoms that help distinguish patients with dementia from those without, and the reliability of brief assessment tests that can be incorporated into primary care practice when appropriate. The purpose of this report is to systematically review the evidence on identifying the signs and symptoms of dementia in undiagnosed patients, and evaluating several brief mental status measures currently being used in VHA. The key questions and scope of this review are the following:

Key Question #1. What signs and symptoms should prompt VA providers to assess cognitive function as part of an initial diagnostic workup for dementia?

Key Question #2. Which measures of cognitive function provide the optimal sensitivity, specificity, and time to completion among the measures available to VA providers?

Key Question #3. What are adverse consequences of using these measures?

Population: Adults without prior diagnosis of dementia.

Measures to be compared: Blessed Orientation-Memory-Concentration (BOMC) Test, Mini-Cog, Montreal Cognitive Assessment (MoCA), General Practitioner Assessment of Cognition (GPCOG), St. Louis University Mental Status (SLUMS) Exam, and Short Test of Mental Status (STMS).

Outcomes: Likelihood for patients to be appropriately diagnosed and treated for dementia; and adverse consequences of assessment, such as depression and anxiety.

Settings: Primary general medicine, mental health, geriatric clinics, specialty clinics, and extended-care settings.

The DSC served as the technical expert panel for guiding topic development and reviewing drafts of the report.

METHODS

We conducted searches in MEDLINE (PubMed), PsychINFO, CINAHL, HAPI, and AGELINE databases for literature published from database inception through July 2009. We obtained additional articles from systematic reviews, reference lists of pertinent studies, narrative reviews, editorials, and from experts in the field. Two reviewers trained in the critical analysis of literature assessed for relevance the abstracts of citations identified from literatures searches. Full-text articles of potentially relevant abstracts were retrieved for further review. We assessed the quality of studies of diagnostic test accuracy using the Quality Assessment of Diagnostic Accuracy Studies (QUADAS) criteria. We compiled a qualitative synthesis of the evidence.

RESULTS

We reviewed 2,394 titles and abstracts from the electronic search, an additional 88 from reference mining, and 57 from an update search of a selected systematic review. We retrieved 310 full-text articles for further review. Of these, we included 18 studies and 1 systematic review in synthesizing evidence for Key Question #1. For Key Question #2, we evaluated the results of 15 diagnostic accuracy studies of the 6 VA cognitive measures. To address Key Question #3, we included 3 cross-sectional studies on the acceptability of dementia screening and diagnostic workup.

KEY QUESTION #1. What signs and symptoms should prompt VA providers to assess cognitive function as part of an initial diagnostic workup for dementia?

Relatively few studies have rigorously evaluated signs and symptoms that may help distinguish people with mild to moderate dementia from non-demented individuals. Subjective memory complaints (SMC) and neuropsychiatric symptoms have been the best studied symptoms.

Epidemiologic studies suggest that SMC – in most cases, elicited with single- or multi-item questionnaires rather than spontaneous – are common in community-living elderly adults. The ability, however, of SMC to discriminate effectively between healthy elderly adults and those with dementia is uncertain. We examined cross-sectional studies comparing rates of SMC between persons with dementia and healthy elderly controls. Patient-reported SMC did not reliably distinguish demented from non-demented individuals. In populations with low rates of dementia, the absence of SMC may have some utility in excluding a diagnosis of dementia. Informant-reported memory complaints may better distinguish demented from non-demented individuals.

A limited body of evidence examined neuropsychiatric symptoms in demented and non-demented individuals. In general, the absence of neuropsychiatric symptoms would not effectively rule out a dementia diagnosis, but the presence of certain symptoms such as apathy, delusions, and/or hallucinations was associated with a dementia diagnosis and may suggest the need for further evaluation. Depression and anxiety were common in demented and non-demented individuals, suggesting the presence of either symptom would not be useful in reliably ruling in or ruling out a diagnosis of dementia.

A very limited body of evidence evaluated sleep disturbance, gait disturbance, and physical exam findings in demented and non-demented individuals. In general, sleep disturbance is a commonly reported symptom in both demented and non-demented individuals, and does not discriminate well the two groups. Gait disturbances are probably useful in distinguishing different subtypes of dementia, but there is little evidence that gait disturbances can clearly distinguish demented from non-demented individuals. Several physical exam findings may be more common in persons with Alzheimer's dementia (AD) than healthy controls. The only finding that was highly specific for AD, however, was impaired sense of touch for perceiving the form of an object (stereognosis), or the form of a letter or number written on the skin (graphesthesia).

KEY QUESTION #2. Which measures of cognitive function provide the optimal sensitivity, specificity, and time to completion among the measures available to VA providers?

All 6 measures available in VA test for recall ability, and 5 of the 6 measures assess executive function by means of a clock drawing test. The assessment of other cognitive domains, such as orientation, abstraction, math, and language skills, varies among the 6 measures.

The Mini-Cog has the shortest administration time of all 6 tests and has been validated in a large sample of the general population. Sensitivity ranged from 76% to 99%, and specificity ranged from 83% to 93% in analyses that excluded patients with mild cognitive impairment (MCI).

The SLUMS test was studied in a VA population and found to have high sensitivity (98-100%) and specificity (98-100%) with adjustment for education. The SLUMS takes longer to administer than other tests. It was developed more recently than the other tests and has not been widely studied.

The STMS has been studied in a primary care setting. The STMS had sensitivity ranging from 86% to 95%, and specificity was highest (93.5%) when cut-off score was adjusted for age. The STMS was evaluated in 2 samples and has not been widely studied.

The GPCOG has been evaluated in a primary care setting, and includes separate sections for patient and informant. The sensitivity of the components ranged from 82% to 98%, but the informant section by itself had low specificity (49-66%). The specificity of the combined score and 2-stage method ranged from 77% to 86%.

The BOMC was evaluated in a bi-racial population sample, and found to misclassify more blacks than whites as impaired. Specificity ranged from 38% to 94%, and sensitivity ranged from 69% to 100%, although the inclusion of patients with previously diagnosed dementia might have inflated the sensitivity in 2 studies.

The MoCA has the longest administration time among the 6 tests, and had low specificity in 2 of 3 studies (35-50%). The MoCA has been evaluated in a memory clinic population but has not been studied in a general practice setting.

KEY QUESTION #3. What are adverse consequences of using these measures?

We found no evidence on adverse effects of the 6 cognitive tests of interest to VA. Three cross-sectional studies assessed the acceptability of dementia screening or diagnostic workup among older adults. The studies reported that high proportions of older adults were unwilling to be routinely tested for memory problems, or to undergo further diagnostic assessment for dementia after having positive results on cognitive screening tests. One survey determined that 80% of respondents wanted to know if they had dementia, but only 57% would agree to routine testing by a physician. Perceived harms included worry about losing insurance, and fear of losing drivers license. The high refusal rates of screening and diagnostic workup indicate the need for further research to understand the psychological burden associated with cognitive tests and assessment for dementia.

EVIDENCE REPORT

BACKGROUND

In 2004, the Office of the Assistant Deputy Under Secretary for Health for Policy and Planning estimated that the total number of Veterans with dementia would be as high as 563,758 in FY 2010.[1] A cost analysis of data from the VA determined that the average annual cost of care for a patient with dementia was $19,522 in FY 1999.[2]

Broad-based dementia screening programs have not been widely advocated given lack of evidence that earlier detection will improve health outcomes.[3, 4] When implemented, screening programs have been associated with high false positive rates, patient hesitation to undergo diagnostic confirmation, and high cost per case identified.[5] Furthermore, several studies have suggested the public is concerned about the implications of dementia screening.[6-8]

The alternative to systematic screening is a case-finding approach in which clinicians initiate diagnostic assessment of dementia when patients and/or their caregivers describe symptoms or present with signs suggestive of dementia. However, with current case-finding approaches, the diagnosis of dementia is often missed in primary care practice.[9-11]

Improving the accuracy of case-finding techniques depends both on an understanding of signs and symptoms that help distinguish patients with dementia from those without, and the reliability of brief assessment tests that can be incorporated into primary care practice when appropriate. Currently, several organizations have issued statements including signs and symptoms that should prompt a diagnostic evaluation for dementia.[12] However, these recommendations are based largely on expert opinion.

One objective of this review, then, is to determine which signs and symptoms help distinguish demented patients from those without dementia. The second objective of this review is to compare the relative accuracy and usability of 6 brief dementia assessment methods available for use in VA.

METHODS

TOPIC DEVELOPMENT

This review was requested by the VHA Dementia Steering Committee (DSC) and commissioned by the Department of Veterans Affairs' Evidence-based Synthesis Program (ESP). The DSC served as the technical expert panel for guiding topic development and reviewing drafts of the report.

In 2007, a workgroup of expert VA clinicians identified 6 brief mental status measures as possible alternatives to the Mini-Mental State Examination (MMSE): Blessed Orientation-Memory-Concentration (BOMC) Test, Mini-Cog, Montreal Cognitive Assessment (MoCA), General Practitioner Assessment of Cognition (GPCOG), St. Louis University Mental Status (SLUMS) Exam, and Short Test of Mental Status (STMS). The MMSE, a widely-used clinical instrument for detecting cognitive impairment, requires payment or permission before it can be reproduced or distributed, under copyright by the Psychological Assessment Resources (PAR). The 6 alternative measures were selected by an internal VA panel on the basis of brevity, applicability in a range of settings including primary care, accuracy in detecting cognitive disturbance, and availability for use in VA clinical and research settings without payment of royalty fees. The instruments are available on an internal VA website: http://vaww.mentalhealth.va.gov/mmse.asp.

The objectives of this review are to address the following questions:

Key Question #1. What signs and symptoms should prompt VA providers to assess cognitive function as part of an initial diagnostic workup for dementia?

Key Question #2. Which measures of cognitive function provide the optimal sensitivity, specificity, and time to completion among the measures available to VA providers?

Key Question #3. What are adverse consequences of using these measures?

These questions were explored within the following contexts:

Population: Adults without prior diagnosis of dementia.

Interventions to be compared: Six specific measures that VA has identified as alternatives to MMSE: BOMC, Mini-Cog, GPCOG, STMS, SLUMS, and MoCA.

Outcomes: Likelihood for patients to be appropriately diagnosed and treated for dementia; and adverse consequences of assessment, such as depression and anxiety.

Settings: Primary general medicine, mental health, geriatric clinics, specialty clinics, and extended-care settings.

SEARCH STRATEGY

We conducted searches in MEDLINE (PubMed), PsychINFO, CINAHL, HAPI, and AGELINE databases for cross-sectional studies comparing demented to non-demented participants, published from database inception through July 2009. Appendix A provides the search strategy in detail. We obtained additional articles from systematic reviews, reference lists of pertinent studies, reviews, editorials, and by consulting experts. All citations were imported into an electronic database (EndNote X2).

STUDY SELECTION

Two reviewers assessed for relevance the abstracts of citations identified from literature searches. Full-text articles of potentially relevant abstracts were retrieved for further review. Each article retrieved was reviewed using the eligibility criteria shown in Appendix B.

Eligible articles had English-language abstracts and provided primary data relevant to the key questions. Eligibility criteria varied depending on the question of interest, as described below.

To evaluate the signs and symptoms of dementia, we determined the prevalence of signs/ symptoms potentially associated with dementia in cross-sectional studies that compared patients with newly diagnosed, mild to moderate dementia with non-demented participants. We excluded studies with only demented individuals or only non-demented individuals, studies that did not provide prevalence data regarding signs and symptoms, and studies that did not use a reference standard to confirm the diagnosis of dementia. Because we were assessing signs and symptoms of prevalent dementia, we excluded studies on signs and symptoms that predicted future dementia.

To evaluate the 6 cognitive tests selected for use in VA, we included diagnostic accuracy studies that compared the performance of the index test against a reference standard for dementia diagnosis, such as DSM-IV. We included studies that compared demented patients with cognitive normal patients, or that included patients with mild cognitive impairment in either the demented or non-demented group. We excluded studies that assessed the performance of the index test for detecting mild cognitive impairment only. We included observational studies on the adverse effects of cognitive assessment.

DATA ABSTRACTION

For each study we abstracted the following: study design, objectives, setting, population characteristics, subject eligibility and exclusion criteria, number of subjects, the standard diagnostic criteria used, and the severity of and type of dementia. For Key Question #1, we additionally abstracted the prevalence of the sign/symptom among demented patients and among non-demented patients. For Key Question #2, we additionally abstracted the proportion of subjects with dementia; the cognitive measure and cut-off score used; the cognitive groups compared; subgroups analyzed (e.g. age, education, race); sensitivity and specificity; the administration time of the test; and any additional test characteristics such as inter-rater reliability, test-retest reliability, and internal consistency. Positive and negative likelihood ratios with 95% confidence intervals were calculated using STATA version 10.1.

QUALITY ASSESSMENT

We assessed the quality of studies using the Quality Assessment of Diagnostic Accuracy Studies (QUADAS) criteria for evaluating diagnostic accuracy studies.[13] Each sign or symptom was considered a diagnostic test, and the QUADAS criteria were used for quality assessment for these studies as well. The QUADAS tool includes 14 criteria that assess applicability, validity, and potential sources of bias, with each item scored as "yes," "no," or "unclear". Appendix C lists the QUADAS criteria in detail. We did not calculate an overall quality score for each study, since the importance of individual items varies according to context, and the use of summary scores for reviews of diagnostic studies is problematic.[14] We noted selected characteristics of studies that may affect quality.

DATA SYNTHESIS

We constructed evidence tables showing the study characteristics and results for all included studies for Key Questions #1 and #2. We critically analyzed studies to compare their characteristics, methods, and findings. We compiled a summary of findings for each key question, and drew conclusions based on qualitative synthesis of the findings.

PEER REVIEW

A draft version of this report was sent to the technical advisory panel and additional peer reviewers. Reviewer comments and our responses are found in Appendix D.

RESULTS

LITERATURE SEARCH

We reviewed 2,394 titles and abstracts from the electronic search, an additional 88 from reference mining, and 57 from conducting an update search of a relevant systematic review.

After applying inclusion/exclusion criteria at the abstract level, we retrieved 310 full-text articles for further review. Of the full-text articles, we rejected 273 that did not meet our inclusion criteria (Figure 1). We included 18 studies and 1 systematic review in synthesizing evidence for key question #1. For key question #2, we evaluated the results of 15 diagnostic accuracy studies of the 6 VA cognitive measures. To address key question #3, we included 3 cross-sectional studies on the acceptability of dementia screening and diagnostic workup.

Figure 1. Literature Flow

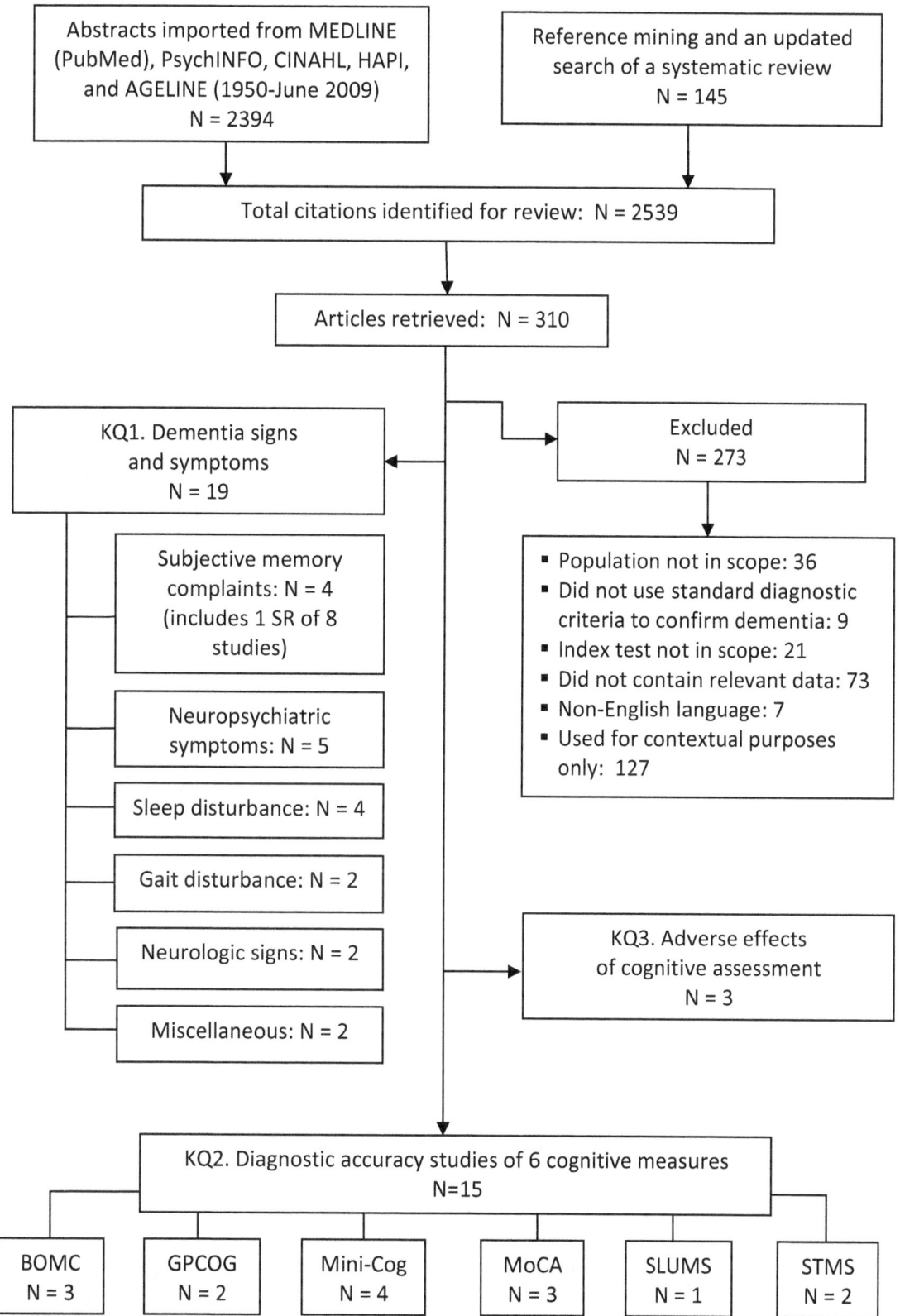

KEY QUESTION #1. What signs and symptoms should prompt VA providers to assess cognitive function as part of an initial diagnostic workup for dementia?

Studies that examined signs and symptoms in demented and non-demented individuals are shown in the table below. The findings for each sign/symptom are described following Table 1.

Table 1. Study characteristics, sensitivity, and specificity of dementia signs and symptoms

Sign/ symptom	N of subjects, setting, country, dementia prevalence, type, and severity (MMSE if available)	Sensitivity of sign/symptom (unless otherwise specified)	Specificity of sign/symptom (unless otherwise specified)	Comments
Subjective memory complaints – self-reported [15]	Total pooled N = 9,148 Meta-analysis of 8 studies, U.S. Largely population based samples Dementia prevalence: 8.8% Severity: NR	Range: 31 – 96%.	Range: 30 – 98%	Good quality review, but methodologic flaws and study heterogeneity limit confidence in pooled results. Many of the included studies had methodologic flaws.
Subjective memory complaints – self-reported [16]	N = 339 Primary care, U.S. Dementia prevalence: 9.7% Type: NR Severity: NR	Self-reported SMC: 15.2% (5/33)	Self-reported SMC: 93.5% (285/305)	Depended on chart documentation of a self-reported symptom – may grossly underestimate the prevalence of the symptom and inflate specificity.
Subjective memory complaints – self-reported [17]	N = 358 Community based sample, U.S. Dementia screen positive (MMSE <25): 31.0% Dementia type: NR CDR < 1: 61.8% CDR 1-3: 23.5% CDR > 3: 14.7%	Self-reported SMC (patients with CDR ≥ 1): 29.5%	Self-reported SMC: 82.2%	Subjects screened with MMSE so prevalence of dementia is higher than would be expected in pure population sample. Prevalence of SMC in patients with CDR = 0.5 (questionable dementia) was 24.8%.
Subjective memory complaints – informant reported [18]	N = 482 Community based sample, U.S. Dementia prevalence: NC Dementia type: AD CDR 0: 32.8% CDR 0.5: 34.2% CDR 1: 33.0%	Self-reported SMC (patients with CDR ≥ 1): 75.3% Informant-reported SMC (patients with CDR ≥ 1): 98.1%	Self-reported SMC (including patients with questionable dementia in control group): 35.6% Self-reported SMC (excluding patients with questionable dementia): 56.3% Informant-reported SMC (excluding patients with questionable dementia): 86.1%	The only study using single question assessment of informant-reported SMC. Self-reported SMC correlated with depressive symptoms.

A Systematic Evidence Review of the Signs and Symptoms of Dementia and Brief Cognitive Tests Available in VA

Sign/ symptom	N of subjects, setting, country, dementia prevalence, type, and severity (MMSE if available)	Sensitivity of sign/symptom (unless otherwise specified)	Specificity of sign/symptom (unless otherwise specified)	Comments
Neuro-psychiatric symptoms [19]	N =1,563 randomly selected from community, Brazil Dementia prevalence: 6.8% AD: N = 60 CIND: N = 25 Randomly selected healthy controls: N = 78 MMSE: 15.5 ± 4.9	Sensitivities AD v CIND + control: Delusion 11.7% (7/60) Hallucination 8.3% (5/60) Agitation/aggression 20% (12/60) Depression 38.3% (23/60) Anxiety 25% (15/60) Elation 5% (3/60) Apathy 53.3% (32/60) Disinhibition 16.7% (10/60) Irritability 23.3% (14/60) Aberrant motor behavior 10% (6/60) Sleep disturbance 38.3% (23/60) Appetite alteration 23.3% (14/60)	Specificities AD v CIND + control: Delusion 100% (103/103) Hallucination 100% (103/103) Agitation/aggression 94.2% (97/103) Depression 87.4% (90/103) Anxiety 89.3% (92/103) Elation 100% (103/103) Apathy 96.1% (99/103) Disinhibition 100% (103/103) Irritability 96.1% (99/103) Aberrant motor behavior 100% (103/103) Sleep disturbance 91.2% (94/103) Appetite alteration 99.0% (102/103)	Dementia patients were older and less well-educated.
Neuro-psychiatric symptoms [20]	N = 682 Cross-sectional substudy of cardiovascular health study, U.S. Patients (at 3 of 4 sites) from pool considered "high-risk" for AD and non-AD dementia Dementia prevalence: 33.4% (24% if risk-screened patients excluded) MCI prevalence: 27.2% Severity: NR	Dementia (%) vs MCI* Delusions 18% (65/362) v 3.1 v 2.4 Hallucinations 10.5% (38/362) v 1.3 v 0.6 Agitation/aggression 30.3% (110/362) v 11.3 v 2.9 Depression 32.3% (117/362) v 20.1 v 7.2 Anxiety 21.5% (78/362) v 9.9 v 5.8 Euphoria 3.1% (11/362) v 0.6 v 0.3 Apathy 35.9% (130/362) v 14.7 v 3.2 Disinhibition 12.7% (46/362) v 3.1 v 0.9 Irritability 27.0% (98/362) v 14.7 v 4.6 Aberrant motor behavior 16% (58/362) v 3.8 v 0.4 Sleep disturbance 27.4% (99/362) v 13.8 v NA Eating disturbance 19.6% (71/362) v 10.4 v NA	Dementia vs MCI: Delusions 96.9% (310/320) Hallucinations 98.7% (316/320) Agitation/aggression 88.7% (284/320) Depression 79.9% (256/320) Anxiety 90.1% (290/320) Euphoria 99.4% (318/320) Apathy 85.3% (273/320) Disinhibition 96.9% (310/320) Irritability 85.3% (273/320) Aberrant motor behavior 96.2% (308/320) Sleep disturbance 86.2% (276/320) Eating disturbance 89.6% (287/320)	Higher dementia prevalence since nearly half the participants had high pre-test probability of cognitive disturbance. Non-demented population data derived from a different cohort.
Neuro-psychiatric symptoms [21]	N = 1002 Community, U.S. Dementia prevalence (MMSE screen positive): 18.4% Predominantly AD and vascular dementia Severity: NR	Sensitivities: Delusions 18.5% (61/329) Hallucinations 13.7% (45/329) Depression 23.7% (78/329) Anxiety 17.0% (56/329) Apathy 27.4% (90/329) Irritability 20.4% (67/329) Agitation/aggression 23.7% (78/329) Disinhibition 9.1% (30/329) Aberrant motor behavior 14.3% (47/329)	Specificities: Delusions 97.0% (653/673) Hallucinations 99.3% (668/673) Depression 92.7% (624/673) Anxiety 93.3% (628/673) Apathy 96.6% (650/673) Irritability 95.1% (640/673) Agitation/aggression 96.9% (652/673) Disinhibition 98.8% (665/673) Aberrant motor behavior 98.4% (662/673)	Population-based design and high participation rates. Subjects screened with MMSE so prevalence of dementia is higher than would be expected in pure population sample.

A Systematic Evidence Review of the Signs and Symptoms of Dementia and Brief Cognitive Tests Available in VA

Sign/ symptom	N of subjects, setting, country, dementia prevalence, type, and severity (MMSE if available)	Sensitivity of sign/symptom (unless otherwise specified)	Specificity of sign/symptom (unless otherwise specified)	Comments
Depression (DSM-IV) [22]	N = 1260 Cross-sectional substudy of general population cohort study, Finland Dementia prevalence: 8.9% Mainly AD and vascular dementia MMSE: 17.0 in those without dementia documented in chart 12.7 in those with dementia documented in chart	32% (36/112)	81.8% (929/1136)	Population-based design and high participation rates are strengths. Study mainly looked at rates of documentation in chart.
Depression [23]	N = 86 Specialty center, U.S. Dementia prevalence: NC Dementia type: NR MMSE/CDR: NR	Mild, moderate or severe depression according to Hamilton Rating Scale for Depression: 40.9%	Mild, moderate or severe depression according to Hamilton Rating Scale for Depression: 88%	
Sleep disturbance [24]	N = 310 Memory clinic, U.S. Dementia prevalence: 50% Type: NR Severity: NR	Poor sleep quality (PSQI > 5): 34.2% (53/155)	Poor sleep quality (PSQI > 5): 40% (62/155)	Subtypes of dementia not reported.
Sleep disturbance [25]	N = 662 Specialty clinic, U.S. Dementia prevalence: NC Dementia type AD MMSE: 19.2 ± 6.2	Subjective sleep problems: 27.6% (71/258)	Subjective sleep problems: 82.7% (320/393)	Non-demented patients self-reported information, while caregivers of demented patients often reported information for demented subgroup.
Sleep disturbance [26]	N = 641 Population-based sample of persons ≥ 81 yo, Sweden Dementia prevalence: NR Type: NR Severity: NR	Subjective sleep disturbance (Comprehensive Psychopathological Rating Scale): 17.8% N not reported	Subjective sleep disturbance: 73.1%	Unclear duration of dementia diagnosis, little information about cohort.

12

Sign/ symptom	N of subjects, setting, country, dementia prevalence, type, and severity (MMSE if available)	Sensitivity of sign/symptom (unless otherwise specified)	Specificity of sign/symptom (unless otherwise specified)	Comments
REM sleep behavior disorder [27]	N = 65 Movement disorder clinic, U.K. Parkinsons Disease Severity: NR	Sensitivity: 77% (10/13)	Specificity: 73% (38/52)	Applicable to Parkinson's dementia only. Unclear proportion of dementia diagnoses that were made retrospectively. Convenience sample. RBD diagnosed with questionnaire, not polysomnography.
Gait disorders [28]	N = 245, age > 65 Specialty clinics, U.K. Dementia prevalence: NC AD, vascular, Parkinsons, and DLB Cambridge Examination for Mental Disorders of the Elderly Cognitive subsection score: Control: 94.0 ± 4.7 AD: 59.0 ± 14.5 Vascular dementia: 61.7 ± 18.3 Parkinsons: 63.9 ± 16.3 DLB: 59.7 ± 15.0	Gait or balance disorder (Tinetti score < 7 or balance score < 22): AD – 10/40 (25%) Vascular dementia – 31/39 (79%) Parkinson's – 43/46 (93%) DLB – 24/32 (75%)	Specificity: 93% (39/42)	Convenience sample. Not clear if reference standard was applied to all controls.
Gait disorders [29]	N = 110 Specialty clinic, U.S. Dementia prevalence: NC Type: AD MMSE: 21/55 mild dementia (CDR 1) 20/55 moderate dementia (CDR 2) 14/55 severe dementia (CDR 3)	Disequilibrium 58% (32/55) Wide-based gait 31% (17/55) Short-stepping gait 35% (19/55) Resistance to passive movement 18% (10/55)	Disequilibrium 64% (35/55) Wide-based gait 85% (47/55) Short-stepping gait 84% (46/55) Resistance to passive movement 98% (1/55)	Convenience sample. Purposive sampling of mild, moderate, and severe dementia. Prevalence of frontal gait disorder correlated with severity of dementia.
Neurologic signs [30]	N = 647, Age > 75 Community, Australia Dementia type: NR Severity: NR	Signs associated with dementia in a regression model (p < .05): rigidity, spasticity, snout/grasp reflex, impaired vibration sense		Major methodologic flaws. Selection criteria, index test, and standard criterion not well described. Large number of variables tested in regression model.

A Systematic Evidence Review of the Signs and Symptoms of Dementia and Brief Cognitive Tests Available in VA

Sign/ symptom	N of subjects, setting, country, dementia prevalence, type, and severity (MMSE if available)	Sensitivity of sign/symptom (unless otherwise specified)	Specificity of sign/symptom (unless otherwise specified)	Comments
Neurologic signs [31]	N = 182 Multi-site (primary care, specialty, and community), U.S. Dementia prevalence: NC Type: AD MMSE: 20.9 ± 5.3	Sensitivities: Release signs – 54.7% (52/95) Olfaction – 20.2% (19/95) Stereognosis† and graphesthesia‡ - 22.1% (21/95) Abnormal gait – 33.7% (32/95)	Specificities: Release signs – 90.8% (79/87) Olfaction – 90.7% (79/87) Stereognosis and graphesthesia – 98.9% (1/87) Abnormal gait – 92.9% (6/87)	Convenience sample. Mean estimated duration of Sx nearly 3 years in dementia group. Not clear if "healthy" defined by self-report or by standard criterion.
Pulse pressure [32]	N = 192 Memory clinic (cases) and community (controls), Korea Dementia prevalence: 63.1% Type: AD MMSE: 16.2 ± 5.8	Mean pulse pressure, cases: 58.9 ± 16.0	Mean pulse pressure, controls: 54.3 ± 11.3	Convenience samples taken from two different populations, with case patients enrolled from a memory clinic.
Driving ability [33]	N = 75 Neurology clinic, U.S. Cross-sectional study from a larger longitudinal study of driving and AD Dementia prevalence: NC MMSE: Mild AD: 21.5 ± 3.9 Very mild AD: 24.9 ± 3.6	Self-reported less than "safe" driving ability: 6% (3/50)	Self-reported less than "safe" driving ability: specificity: 100% (24/24)	Not a population-based sample. Focused mainly on correlation between self-rated and on-road driving performance in demented patients.

*Controls taken from a different cohort, therefore figures represent comparison of demented patients to those with MCI

†Stereognosis = the ability to perceive the form of an object by using the sense of touch

‡Graphesthesia = the ability to recognize a number or letter written on the skin by the sensation of touch

Abbreviations: AD = Alzheimer's disease, CIND = Cognitively impaired non-demented, DLB = Dementia with Lewy bodies, MCI = Mild cognitive impairment, NC = cannot be calculated, PSQI = Pittsburgh Sleep Quality Index, SMC = subjective memory complaints, Sx = symptoms

14

Subjective memory complaints

Summary of findings (Table 1)

Epidemiologic studies suggest subjective memory complaints (SMC) – in most cases elicited with single- or multi-item questionnaires, rather than spontaneous – are common in community-living elderly adults.[34, 35] The ability, however, of subjective memory complaints to discriminate effectively between healthy elderly adults and those with dementia is uncertain. We examined cross-sectional studies comparing rates of SMC between persons with dementia and healthy elderly controls.

Conclusions from this body of evidence should be tempered by methodologic flaws in some of the studies, as well as variability across studies in populations included and methods used for memory complaint elicitation. We found patient-reported SMC did not reliably distinguish demented from non-demented individuals. Patient-reported SMC were poorly sensitive for detecting dementia and only moderately specific. In populations with low prevalence of dementia, the absence of SMC may have some utility in excluding a diagnosis of dementia given its relatively high negative predictive value in these settings. Informant-reported memory complaints may better distinguish demented from non-demented individuals.

Detailed description

One recently published systematic review found 8 cross-sectional studies which compared elicited patient-reported SMC in demented and non-demented persons.[15] All studies were community-based and ranged in size from 156 to 3,220 participants. A number of the included studies had substantial flaws which reduce the strength of conclusions that can be drawn from this body of literature. Three studies established a dementia diagnosis using a widely-accepted gold standard.[36-38] One of the studies used a less widely-accepted cognitive evaluation,[39] and another study used an informant interview to establish a diagnosis.[40] Three of the studies used only brief assessment methods to validate the diagnosis of dementia.[41-43] Because of significant heterogeneity among studies, the pooled results cannot be used with any degree of confidence.

Of the 3 studies that used a widely-accepted gold standard to establish a dementia diagnosis,[36-38] one was mainly a study of different subtypes of mild cognitive impairment (MCI) and the number of patients with dementia was very low.[38] Tobiansky, et al.[36] and St. John, et al.[37] both examined large community-based samples, but used different methods for eliciting SMC: 1 study used a 9-item questionnaire,[36] while the other study simply asked whether participants had had memory loss during the past year.[37]

We found several more recent studies that were not included in the Mitchell review. One community-based study found a very low sensitivity of 15.2%, but a relatively high specificity of 93.5%.[16] However, these rates were likely a reflection of the method of SMC ascertainment, which relied on retrospective chart review. A multi-site primary care study of patients with largely mild dementia found patient-reported SMC also did not distinguish well between demented and non-demented participants.[17] Of note, investigators did find greater discrepancies between patient interview results and chart notes among patients with more severe dementia.

In contrast to patient-reported SMC, a small body of evidence suggests informant-reported SMC may better distinguish demented from non-demented individuals. One study of patients with mild and very mild Alzheimer's type dementia (AD) found informant complaints of memory loss (using a single question assessment) more reliably correlated with dementia than patient complaints (sensitivity of informant complaints 98.1%, specificity 86.1%).[18] Furthermore, patient-reported SMC did not predict future onset of dementia, whereas informant-reported SMC were associated with an increased risk of future dementia, a finding similar to a prior longitudinal study.[44] Patient complaints of memory loss in this study were closely associated with depressive symptomatology, findings that corroborate those of older studies.[44, 45]

Table 2 uses data from 2 of the self-reported SMC studies and the informant-reported memory complaint study to compare positive and negative predictive values in hypothetical populations with differing prevalence rates of dementia. All 3 studies suggest in populations with low rates of dementia, the lack of memory complaints may help exclude a dementia diagnosis, and the lack of informant memory complaints may most reliably exclude a diagnosis of dementia.

Table 2. Sensitivity, specificity, and predictive values of memory complaints in selected studies

Population	Sensitivity	Specificity	Prevalence assumption	Positive Predictive Value	Negative Predictive Value
Community sample [37]	58.0%	76.0%	10% 50% 75%	21.2% 70.7% 87.9%	94.2% 64.4% 37.6%
Community sample [36]	46.0%	97.0%	10% 50% 75%	63.1% 93.9% 97.9%	94.2% 64.2% 37.5%
Community sample – informant-reported memory complaints [18]	98.1%	86.1%	10% 50% 75%	43.8% 87.5% 94.6%	99.7% 97.7% 82.7%

A brief informant questionnaire, which combines 3 questions on informant-reported memory complaints with 5 questions covering other domains, including judgment and financial management, has been evaluated in demented and non-demented individuals. The questionnaire – the AD8 – discriminated well between demented and non-demented individuals (area under the curve 0.92; 95% CI 0.88 – 0.95).[46] The same authors later compared the utility of informant-administered to patient-administered AD8 and found both distinguished demented from non-demented individuals, but the informant-administered questionnaire performed better.[47]

Neuropsychiatric symptoms

Summary of findings

We found 3 community-based studies which used the Neuropsychiatric Inventory (NPI)[48] to compare neuropsychiatric symptoms in demented and non-demented persons. In general, neuropsychiatric symptoms were poorly sensitive but moderately to highly specific for dementia. Apathy was the most common neuropsychiatric symptom reported in demented persons and was present much less frequently in non-demented persons. Depression and anxiety were common in both groups, suggesting the presence of either symptom would not be useful in reliably ruling in or ruling out a diagnosis of dementia.

Detailed description

One well-conducted study included elderly residents of Cache County, Utah, and used a modified, more sensitive version of the Mini-Mental State Exam (MMSE) to identify a subpopulation at higher risk for dementia; and also included a randomly selected MMSE screen negative population.[21] All participants underwent a comprehensive cognitive assessment and were categorized as demented or non-demented according to DSM-IV criteria. The prevalence of dementia (18.4%) in this study reflects the use of MMSE as an initial screen and is higher than would be expected in the general population. Neuropsychiatric symptoms were more common in demented than non-demented individuals and 61% of demented individuals had had at least one behavorial symptom in the last month. Over 1 in 4 people with dementia were reported to display apathy, compared to less than 1 in 20 non-demented people. Depression was least helpful in distinguishing healthy elderly controls (specificity 92.7%).

Another study used a subsample of data from the Cardiovascular Health Study, and nearly half the participants had a high pre-test probability of cognitive dysfunction, which was reflected in the study's high prevalence of dementia (33.4%).[20] The study cohort included persons with dementia and mild cognitive impairment (MCI), but the non-demented comparison group was derived from a separate cohort in which sampling methods may have been different. Therefore, we only report sensitivity and specificity data comparing persons with dementia to persons with MCI. As expected, the specificities were lower, suggesting a higher likelihood of neuropsychiatric symptom presence in persons with MCI than healthy controls.

A community-based Brazilian study with a lower prevalence of dementia also had largely similar findings, but findings from this study may be less generalizable to VA populations in the United States.[19]

One population-based study focused on accuracy of dementia documentation in medical records of persons with and without dementia, but included the prevalence rates of depression in demented and non-demented people.[22] Similar to other studies, depression had a low sensitivity and specificity for dementia (32.0% and 81.8%, respectively). These results were similar to a small, older study of depression in demented and non-demented persons.[23]

Sleep disturbance

We found 4 studies comparing the frequency of sleep disturbance in patients with and without dementia. One of these studies compared the frequency of REM Sleep Behavior Disorder (RBD) in a convenience sample of Parkinson's disease patients with and without dementia, and is not applicable to patients with other types of dementia.[27]

The remaining 3 studies examined sleep disturbance in persons with and without dementia, mainly of Alzheimer's type.[24-26] In general, sleep disturbance is a commonly reported symptom in both demented and non-demented individuals, and does not discriminate the groups well. In fact, 2 of the studies found a higher prevalence of sleep disturbance complaints in non-demented than in demented persons.[24, 26] Results from the third study are more difficult to interpret because sleep disturbance questionnaires were completed by caregivers of demented participants, whereas non-demented participants in the control group completed the questionnaires themselves.[25] The body of evidence is limited by differences in definition of sleep disturbance, disparate patient populations and settings, and limited direct applicability to primary care settings.

Gait disturbance

Summary of findings

Only 2 studies have compared gait disturbance frequency in persons with and without dementia. Gait disturbances are probably useful in distinguishing different subtypes of dementia, but there is little evidence that gait disturbances can clearly distinguish demented from non-demented individuals.

Detailed description

Early presence of gait disturbance had been thought an uncommon finding in AD and, in fact, is cited as a factor negatively associated with the diagnosis in the NINCDS-ADRDA criteria for AD.[49] One small study examined the prevalence of various types of gait disturbance in patients with various stages of AD and in a poorly defined control population.[29] They found that cautious gait was a common finding in both early stage AD and in healthy controls. Findings consistent with frontal gait disturbance, on the other hand, were more common with increasing severity of disease, but very uncommon in healthy participants.

The second study compared gait and balance disorder frequency between persons with different dementia subtypes and also to healthy controls.[28] Not surprisingly, gait and balance disorders were significantly more common in persons with vascular, Lewy-body, and Parkinson's dementia than in persons with AD. Gait and balance disturbance was slightly more prevalent in persons with AD than in controls (odds ratio 4, 95% CI 1.1 – 17).

Neurologic signs

Several physical exam findings may be more common in persons with AD than healthy controls. In one study using a convenience sample of persons with mild AD, release signs, olfactory deficit, impaired sense of touch, and an abnormal gait were all more common in persons with AD.[31] The only finding, however, that was highly specific for AD was stereognosis (the ability to perceive the form of an object by using the sense of touch) and graphesthesia (the ability to recognize writing on the skin purely by the sensation of touch), with sensitivity of 22.1% and specificity of 98.9%. None of the signs were very sensitive for dementia, though release signs were present in over half the participants with AD (sensitivity 54.7%).

Another study using a population-based sample also examined a number of neurologic signs and found that rigidity, spasticity, and frontal release signs were associated with dementia in a regression model.[30] The study findings were somewhat consistent with the aforementioned study; however, the study evaluated a large number of signs in a regression model and it is possible some of the findings reflect a chance finding given the multiple variables examined.

Miscellaneous

The final 2 studies provide interesting preliminary data but are not part of a robust enough body of evidence to draw firm conclusions. One study examined the relationship between pulse pressure and AD, and found higher mean pulse pressure among persons with AD compared with their non-demented counterparts (58.9 vs. 54.3, $p < 0.05$). The result suggests higher pulse pressure was associated with increased white matter changes.[32] However, the study has some methodologic flaws, the most important being the case and control groups were derived from different populations.

One study focused primarily on the correlation between self-reported and on-road driving performance, but did examine self-reported rating of "safe" driving ability in patients with and without dementia.[33] Most demented persons rated themselves as safe drivers even though informants and driving instructors were much less likely to rate their driving as safe. The sensitivity of less than safe driving ability for identifying dementia is, not surprisingly, very low.

KEY QUESTION #2. Which measures of cognitive function provide the optimal sensitivity, specificity, and time to completion, among the measures available to VA providers?

Summary of findings

All 6 measures available in VA test for recall ability, and 5 of the 6 measures assess executive function by means of a clock drawing test. The assessment of other cognitive domains, such as orientation, abstraction, and aphasia, varies among the 6 measures.

The Mini-Cog has the shortest administration time of all 6 tests and has been validated in a large sample of the general population. Sensitivity ranged from 76% to 99%, and specificity ranged from 83% to 93% in analyses that excluded patients with MCI.

The SLUMS test was studied in a VA population and found to have high sensitivity (98-100%) and specificity (98-100%) with adjustment for education. The SLUMS takes longer to administer than other tests. It was developed more recently than the other tests and has not been widely studied.

The STMS has been studied in a primary care setting. The STMS had sensitivity ranging from 86% to 95%, and specificity was highest (93.5%) when cut-off score was adjusted for age. The STMS was evaluated in 2 samples and has not been widely studied.

The GPCOG has been evaluated in a primary care setting, and includes separate sections for patient and informant. The sensitivity of the components ranged from 82% to 98%, but the informant section by itself had low specificity (49-66%). The specificity of the combined score and 2-stage method ranged from 77% to 86%.

The BOMC was evaluated in a bi-racial population sample, and found to misclassify more blacks than whites as impaired. Specificity ranged from 38% to 94%, and sensitivity ranged from 69% to 100%, although the inclusion of patients with previously diagnosed dementia might have inflated the sensitivity in 2 studies.

The MoCA has the longest administration time among the 6 tests, and had low specificity in 2 of 3 studies (35-50%). The MoCA has been evaluated in a memory clinic population, but has not been studied in a general practice setting.

Table 3 summarizes the strengths and limitations of each test. Detailed findings are provided in the pages that follow.

Table 3. Pros and cons of 6 brief mental status measures available for use in VA

Test	Pros	Cons
BOMC	• Studied in a general population sample and 2 specialty clinic settings	• Low specificity (38-77%) in 2 of 4 studies • Race and education biases in 1 study
GPCOG	• Studied in a primary care setting • Education bias found absent • The combined score and 2-stage method had higher sensitivity and specificity than patient and informant sections separately	• Informant section alone has low specificity (49-66%)
Mini-Cog	• Shortest administration time (2-4 minutes) • Studied in a general population sample • High specificity (83-93%) in studies that excluded MCI from comparator group • Education and language/race biases found absent in U.S. samples	• May be inappropriate for populations with extremely low levels of education or literacy
MoCA	• Studied in a memory clinic population • High sensitivity (94-100%)	• Longest administration time (10-15 minutes) • Low specificity (35-50%) in 2 of 3 studies
SLUMS	• Studied in a VA geriatric clinic population • High sensitivity and specificity (98-100%) • Adjusts cut-off score for education	• Longer administration time (7 minutes) • Evaluated in only 1 study
STMS	• Studied in a primary care setting • Shorter administration time (5 minutes) • High specificity (93.5%) using age-adjusted cutoff scores	• Evaluated in 2 studies

Detailed description

The literature search identified 16 primary studies that assessed the test performance of one or more of the 6 brief cognitive assessments against a standard criterion for diagnosing dementia. Table 4 shows the study characteristics and the test performance results for each cognitive measure. Positive and negative likelihood ratios were calculated using the reported results for sensitivity and specificity, with the exception of 1 study,[50] for which sensitivity and specificity results were derived from a systematic review compiled in 2003 for the U.S. Preventive Services Task Force (USPSTF).[51]

The BOMC test was assessed in 4 studies reported in 6 publications,[50-55] the GPCOG in 2 studies,[56, 57] the Mini-Cog in 3 studies,[58-60] the MoCA in 3 studies,[61-63] SLUMS in 1 study,[64] and STMS in 2 studies.[65, 66]

The cognitive measures were studied in a variety of populations, including primary care, specialty clinics, and residential care/assisted living facilities. The prevalence of dementia varied with study setting (Table 4). Prevalence is not shown for studies that used a constructed sample (e.g. dementia cases matched 1:1 with controls) or that recruited subjects from heterogeneous settings. The prevalence of dementia in Table 4 is defined as the proportion of demented patients in the analyzed sample.

In some studies, subjects with MCI were excluded from the analysis.[58, 60, 61, 64] In other studies, subjects with MCI were included in the non-demented comparison group,[60] or were combined with dementia patients for the assessment of test performance.[62] The inclusion of subjects with MCI in the analysis could negatively affect the operating characteristics of the index test. Combining MCI with dementia would decrease sensitivity if MCI patients were more likely than dementia patients to be misclassified as unimpaired. Conversely, including MCI in the non-demented group would decrease specificity if MCI patients were more likely than cognitively normal subjects to be misclassified as demented.

Table 4. Study characteristics and test performance results for the BOMC, GPCOG, Mini-Cog, MoCA, SLUMS, and STMS

Sample/setting (Reference)	Dementia (%)	Comparison	N total	Cut-off Score	Sens.	Spec.	+LR (95%CI)	-LR (95% CI)
BOMC								
Population sample*[52]	16.9	Black race only: demented v. non-demented	83	11	1.0	0.382	1.56 (1.27-1.91)	0.0881 (0.0057-1.37)
	3.7	White race only: demented v. non-demented	81	11	1.0	0.785	3.95 (2.27-6.88)	0.161 (0.012-2.15)
Memory clinic†‡[53]	83.3	Combined dementias v. normal	282	7/6	0.91	0.63	2.52 (1.72-3.69)	0.14 (0.0883-0.222)
				10/9	0.83	0.77	3.55 (2.11-5.97)	0.222 (0.161-0.307)
Neurology clinic*†‡[54]	33.1	Combined dementias v. normal	133	10/11	0.886	0.944	15.8 (6.69-37.2)	0.12 (0.0527-0.275)
Mixed settings†§[50, 51]	||	Combined dementias v. normal	321	NR	0.69	0.9	7 (4.06-12.1)	0.346 (0.279-0.428)
GPCOG								
General practice: patients aged 75+, and patients aged 50-74 with memory complaints[56]	29.1	Patient section only; demented v. non-demented	282	7/8	0.82	0.7	2.72 (2.15-3.45)	0.261 (0.164-0.417)
		Informant section only	202	4/5	0.89	0.66	2.62 (2.06-3.34)	0.155 (0.0718-0.333)
		Combined score	202	10/11	0.82	0.83	4.85 (3.3-7.12)	0.224 (0.131-0.384)
		Two-stage method	246	---	0.85	0.86	6.14 (4.18-9.02)	0.177 (0.103-0.306)
Mixed settings†¶[57]	||	Patient section only; definite dementia v. normal (excludes MCI)	118	<=7	0.982	0.672	2.95 (2.06-4.22)	0.0259 (0.0037-0.182)
		Informant section only	80	<=4	0.942	0.491	1.82 (1.24-2.66)	0.114 (0.0351-0.367)
		Combined score; definite dementia v. normal (excludes MCI)	80	<=10	0.981	0.774	4.09 (2.03-8.23)	0.0239 (0.0034-0.169)
Mini-Cog								
Population sample[58]	6.4	Demented v. normal (excludes MCI)	1119	2/3	0.76	0.89	6.95 (5.61-8.62)	0.265 (0.175-0.402)
Residential care/assisted living, without history of dementia†¶#[60]	37.7	Dementia v. (MCI + no cognitive impairment)	146	2/3	0.87	0.54	1.89 (1.48-2.41)	0.236 (0.115-0.484)
Mixed settings; enriched in ethnic minorities, demented patients†[59]	||	Combined dementias v. normal (excludes MCI)	300	2/3	0.969	0.828	5.65 (3.92-8.14)	0.0377 (0.0159-0.0897)
MoCA								
Memory clinic†[61]	72.7 48††	Dementia v. non-demented (excludes MCI)	44	<26	0.94	0.5	1.88 (1.06-3.32)	0.125 (0.0291-0.536)

A Systematic Evidence Review of the Signs and Symptoms of Dementia and Brief Cognitive Tests Available in VA

Sample/setting (Reference)	Dementia (%)	Comparison	N total	Cut-off Score	Sens.	Spec.	+LR (95%CI)	-LR (95% CI)
Mixed settings†**[62]	||	Combined (dementia + MCI) v. normal	118	<=26	0.97	0.35	1.51 (1.27-1.79)	0.0647 (0.0091-0.46)
Patients with history of mild dementia v. controls†[63]	||	Mild AD v. normal (excludes MCI)	183	26	1.0	0.87	7.24 (4.33-12.1)	0.0062 (3.9e-04-0.098)
SLUMS								
VA-GRECC patients aged 60+¶[64]	16.5 12.6††	Education <HS: Dementia v. normal (excludes MCI)	164	19.5	1.0	0.98	38.7 (13.7-109)	0.0183 (0.0012-0.286)
	15.4 11.3††	Education >=HS: Dementia v. normal (excludes MCI)	358	21.5	0.98	1.0	592 (37.1-9442)	0.0268 (0.0055-0.13)
STMS								
Newly diagnosed dementia v. controls in primary care†[66]	||	Dementia v. normal (excludes MCI)	248	<29	0.864	0.884	7.45 (4.67-11.9)	0.154 (0.096-0.248)
		By age: 60-69: 30 70-79: 29 80-89: 28 >90: 27			0.864	0.935	13.2 (7.01-25)	0.146 (0.091-0.234)
Patients with history of dementia v. non-demented controls from a neurology clinic¶[65]	||	Combined dementias v. no dementia (excludes MCI)	180	<=29	0.92	0.914	10.7 (5.5-20.8)	0.088 (0.0431-0.18)
		AD v. no dementia (excludes MCI)	160		0.955	0.914	11.1 (5.71-21.6)	0.049 (0.0162-0.148)
		Aged 60+ only: Combined dementias v. no dementia (excludes MCI)	109		0.947	0.879	7.82 (3.11-19.6)	0.0599 (0.0229-0.157)

* Sample may have included prevalent dementia; sensitivity may be overestimated.
† May not be applicable to primary care populations.
‡ Unclear whether clinic patients were randomly or consecutively sampled.
§ Sensitivity and specificity were calculated in the USPSTF 2003 report[51] based on an AHCPR 1996 meta-analysis.[55]
|| Mixed clinic/community or constructed sample. Prevalence could not be calculated.
¶ Interpretation of index test and reference standard were not fully blinded.
# Non-demented comparison group includes subjects with mild cognitive impairment.

** Subjects with dementia and MCI are compared with cognitively normal subjects.
†† Prevalence of dementia in the total sample that comprised patients with dementia, MCI, and no cognitive impairment. MCI patients were otherwise excluded from the results shown.

Abbreviations: +LR = Positive Likelihood Ratio; -LR = Negative Likelihood Ratio; AD = Alzheimer's Disease; BOMC = Blessed Orientation-Memory-Concentration Test; GPCOG = General Practitioner Assessment of Cognition; MCI = Mild Cognitive Impairment; MoCA = Montreal Cognitive Assessment; Sens. = Sensitivity; SLUMS = St. Louis University Mental Status Exam; Spec. = Specificity; STMS = Short Test of Mental Status

Table 5 on the following page provides descriptive characteristics of the 6 tests, including the time to administer and the cognitive domains assessed.[67] All 6 measures test for recall ability, and assessment for executive function by means of a clock drawing test is a component in all measures except the BOMC. The assessment of other cognitive domains, such as orientation, abstraction, math, and language skills, varies among the 6 measures.

Table 5 also shows characteristics of the tests that were reported in some but not all studies. These include inter-rater reliability; test-retest reliability; internal consistency; and the effects of education, race, and language on test performance. Among the 6 measures, only the Mini-Cog and BOMC were examined for differences by race or language in a biracial or multi-ethnic sample.

In addition, Table 5 displays the sensitivity, specificity, positive likelihood ratio, and negative likelihood ratio from a selected study for each cognitive measure. These representative studies were selected based on applicability to the settings that the samples were drawn from: the general population in the case of the BOMC and Mini-Cog; primary care or a geriatric clinic in the case of the GPCOG, SLUMS, and STMS; and a memory clinic population in the case of the MoCA.

Table 5. Cognitive domains, biases, and other characteristics of BOMC, GPCOG, Mini-Cog, MoCA, SLUMS, and STMS

	BOMC	GPCOG	Mini-Cog	MoCA	SLUMS	STMS
Cognitive domain						
Orientation (e.g. time/place)	X	X		X	X	X
Registration/recall	X	X	X	X	X	X
Remote memory					X	
Praxis, visuospatial		X	X	X	X	X
Aphasia, verbal fluency				X		X
Attention	X			X	X	X
Abstraction				X	X	X
Executive function		X	X	X	X	X
Biases detected						
Education bias	Yes[52,53]	No[56,57]	No[59,68]	Yes*[62]	No[64]	Yes[66]
Language/race bias	Yes[52]	---	No[59,68]	---	---	Yes†[65]
Performance results from selected studies‡	53	56	58	61	64	66
Sensitivity	0.83	Patient only: 0.82 / Two-stage: 0.85	0.76	0.94	<HS: 1.0 / HS+: 0.98	Age-based cutoff: 0.86
Specificity	0.77	0.7 / 0.86	0.89	0.5	0.98 / 1.0	0.935
+LR (95%CI)	3.55 (2.11-5.97)	2.72 (2.2-3.5) / 6.14 (4.2-9.0)	6.95 (5.6-8.6)	1.88 (1.0-3.3)	38.7 (13.7-109) / 592 (37.1-9442)	13.2 (7.0-25)
-LR (95%CI)	0.222 (0.161-0.307)	0.261 (0.16-0.42) / 0.177 (0.10-0.31)	0.265 (0.18-0.40)	0.125 (0.03-0.54)	0.0183 (0.001-0.29) / 0.0268 (0.006-0.13)	0.146 (0.09-0.23)
Other characteristics						
Time to administer, mean or range (min)	4-6	Patient: 2-5 / Informant: 1-3	2-4	10-15	7	5
Inter-rater reliability	Adequate[53,54]	Adequate[56]	Adequate[59]	---	---	---
Test-retest reliability	---	Adequate[56]	---	Adequate[63]	---	---
Internal consistency	---	Adequate[56]	---	Adequate[63]	---	---

* The effect of education on the MoCA was correctable by the inclusion of a 1-point education correction for individuals with 12 or fewer years of education.[62]

† Study authors note that a severe language disturbance would preclude use of the STMS. The test could be administered with the help of interpreters to patients who do not speak English.

‡ A representative study for each cognitive measure was selected based on applicability to the setting that the sample was drawn from: the general population in the case of the Mini-Cog; primary care or a geriatric clin c for the GPCOG, SLUMS, and STMS; and a memory clinic population for the BOMC and the MoCA.

Abbreviations: <HS = less than high school education; HS+ = high school or more education.

**A Systematic Evidence Review of the Signs and Symptoms
of Dementia and Brief Cognitive Tests Available in VA**
        Evidence-based Synthesis Program

BOMC

The BOMC is a 6-item measure derived from the Blessed Information-Memory-Concentration Test.[69] The items are weighted for a total maximum score of 28, and include current date (month, year) and time, counting backwards from 20 to 1, reciting the months of the year in reverse order, and recalling a previously repeated 5-element address.[50] Test-retest reliability of the BOMC was assessed and found adequate in 2 studies.[53, 54] The administration time is 4 to 6 minutes.

The BOMC was assessed in a population-based sample, a memory clinic, a neurology clinic, and in a study with mixed settings (Table 4). Two studies used a cutoff score of 11 (11 or more errors on the weighted 28-point scale indicates impairment),[52, 54] but the cut-off score of 10/9 (given as best score for demented group/worst score for non-demented group) yielded the maximum results for both sensitivity (83%) and specificity (77%) in a study of patients in a memory clinic.[53] Although the sensitivity of the BOMC was found to be 100% in the population-based study,[52] this result may be inflated due to the inclusion of subjects with pre-existing dementia in the sample.

In a population-based subsample from the Established Populations for Epidemiologic Studies of the Elderly (EPESE) cohort, the BOMC was found to misclassify a greater proportion of Africans Americans as demented compared with whites.[52] Specificity was only 38.2% for blacks, compared with 78.5% for whites in this study. Less educated subjects were more likely to be classified as impaired, and the effect of education did not vary by race. The lack of adjustment for education in this study limits interpretation of the observed racial differences. Other studies have reported an association between race and cognitive test scores that persists after controlling for education, suggesting that additional factors such as socioeconomic status, comorbidity, health habits, and social factors, may contribute to the observed racial differences.[70]

GPCOG

The GPCOG contains separate sections for patient and informant. The patient section includes items testing time orientation (3 points, including a clock drawing test), awareness of a news story within the previous week (1 point), and recall of a name and an address (5 points). The informant section includes 6 items that ask an informant to make a comparison between the participant's current function and that from a few years ago. The cognitive and informant sections can be scored separately, together, or sequentially. In the sequential or 2-stage method, the informant section is not required for participants who score >8 (considered cognitively intact) or <5 (considered impaired). For participants who score 5 to 8 (inclusive) on the cognitive section, scores of <=3 on the informant section indicate cognitive impairment.[56]

The GPCOG was assessed in a primary care setting[56] and in subjects recruited through various settings including memory clinics, an Alzheimer's respite program, and other clinics.[57] In the first study, 67 general practitioners in 4 regional divisions in Australia administered the GPCOG to 283 patients aged 75 and older, as well as community-dwelling patients aged 50 to 74 with memory complaints. The prevalence of dementia in the sample was 29.1%. The components of the GPCOG were assessed separately and in combination: patient section only, informant section only, combined score from patient and informant sections, and the 2-stage method. The sensitivity of each ranged from 82% to 89%. The specificity was lower for the informant section only (66%), and the patient section only (70%), compared with the combined score (83%) or 2-stage method (86%). In the study of mixed settings, the sensitivity of the individual or combined sections was higher, ranging from 94.2% to 98.2%; but the specificity was lower: 49% for the informant section, 67.2% for the patient section, and 77.4% for the combined score.[57]

Mini-Cog

The Mini-Cog combines 2 cognitive tasks (3-item word memory and clock drawing) with a sequential scoring method; and was developed in a community sample that overrepresented dementia cases, persons of low education and nonwhite ethnicity, and non-English speakers.[68] We identified 3 studies that assessed the operating characteristics of the Mini-Cog.[58-60] In each of these studies, the results of the Mini-Cog were derived from longer tests that were administered to determine whether the minimum data elements that make up the Mini-Cog would perform as well as or better than the longer, more complex diagnostic tests. The operating characteristics of the Mini-Cog by itself may differ in practice from the research studies included in this review.

Of the 6 VA measures, the Mini-Cog takes the least time to administer (2 to 4 minutes) and has been validated in a large (N=1119), age-stratified, random sample of the general population aged 65 and older (mean age 73.1). The prevalence of dementia in the sample was 6.4%, and the sensitivity and specificity of the Mini-Cog were 0.76 and 0.89, respectively.[58]

In a sample that had proportionally more demented patients (62%)[59] than in the general population (6.4%),[58] the Mini-Cog had higher sensitivity (97% v. 76%) but similar specificity (83% v. 89%). No association was found between education or language on Mini-Cog test performance in a study that included ethnic minorities in the U.S., although both education and language were significantly associated with MMSE test performance in the same sample.[68] In a study of adults aged 65+ in residential care and assisted living facilities who did not have a chart-documented diagnosis of dementia, 37.7% of residents met criteria for probable dementia using DSM-IV criteria. The sensitivity of the Mini-Cog in this sample was 87% and the specificity was 54%.[60] This study included subjects with MCI in the non-demented comparator group, potentially causing a decrease in specificity.

Studies of the Mini-Cog among ethnic minority groups with mixed linguistic and educational backgrounds found that the effects of low education and literacy on the accuracy of the Mini-Cog were weak or absent.[59, 68] In one study, Asian Americans constituted 48% of the sample, African Americans 22%, Hispanics 17%, and white non-Hispanic 7%. The mean years of education were 11.5 among normal subjects, 10.4 among subjects with MCI, and 8.5 among demented subjects in this study.[59] The Mini-Cog performed less accurately in a study of elderly with low education in Brazil, of whom 76% had less than 5 years of schooling and 25% were illiterate.[71] Given that the Mini-Cog was developed to facilitate cognitive screening in primary care settings in first-world countries, the authors of the Mini-Cog suggest that in populations with extremely low levels of education or literacy, informant-based screening or individualized function-based screening might be preferable to the use of cognitive screening tests.[72]

MoCA

The MoCA is a 1-page, 30-point test, and has the longest administration time (10 to 15 minutes) among the 6 tests. Short-term memory recall is assessed by 2 learning trials of 5 nouns and delayed recall after approximately 5 minutes. Visuospatial tasks include a clock drawing task and a 3-dimensional cube copy. Multiple aspects of executive functions are assessed using an alternation task adapted from the Trail Making B task, a phonemic fluency task, and a 2-item verbal abstraction task. Attention, concentration, and working memory are evaluated using a sustained attention task, a serial subtraction task, and digits forward and backward. Language is assessed using a 3-item confrontation naming task with low-familiarity animals (lion, camel, rhinoceros), repetition of 2 syntactically complex sentences, and the aforementioned fluency task. Finally, orientation to time and place is evaluated.[63] The tests, along with instructions for administering and scoring, are available in 30 languages.[73]

Three studies evaluated the test performance of the MoCA.[61-63] One was a prospective study of 67 consecutive patients seen in a memory clinic. In this sample, 48% were determined to have dementia, 34% had MCI, and 12% had an identifiable psychiatric illness that explained subjective memory complaints or had no objective evidence of memory loss.[61] The other 2 studies recruited subjects from mixed settings[62] or used a case-control sample,[63] and prevalence could not be determined. The MoCA has not been validated in a primary care population or a sample representative of the general population.

Although the sensitivity of the MoCA was high (94% to 100%), the specificity of the MoCA was low, ranging from 35% to 50% in 2 of the 3 studies. Individuals with <=12 years of education performed significantly worse on the MoCA (p<0.05). The effect of education, however, was correctable by the inclusion of a 1-point education correction for individuals with 12 years or less of education.[62]

SLUMS

The SLUMS examination is a 30-point, 11-item scale that includes tasks corresponding to attention, numeric calculation, immediate and delayed recall, animal naming, digit span, clock drawing, figure recognition/size differentiation, and immediate recall of facts from a paragraph.[64] The average administration time is 7 minutes.

The SLUMS test was studied in a population of 702 U.S. Veterans aged 60+ in a VA geriatric clinic.[64] The prevalence of dementia in the total sample, including subjects with MCI, was 11.6%. The study stratified subjects by level of education, and determined that the optimal cutoff score was 19.5 for subjects with less than high school education and 21.5 for subjects with high school or more education. Sensitivity and specificity were both high (98% to 100%) with this adjustment for education level.

STMS

The STMS is a 38-point, 8-item scale that tests orientation, attention, immediate recall, arithmetic, abstraction, construction, information, and delayed (approximately 3 minutes) recall.[66] The administration time is approximately 5 minutes.

The STMS was assessed in 2 studies that used a constructed sample of demented patients and non-demented controls. In one study, the demented group included 87 outpatients with mild to moderate severity and mean duration of 3.26 years, ranging from newly diagnosed to 10.3 years.[65] Ninety-three non-demented controls were recruited from consecutive patients who came to the neurologic practice for consultation during a 10-week period. Using a cutoff score of <=29, the sensitivity and specificity of the STMS were high in this study, but generalizability to the primary care setting is limited.

**A Systematic Evidence Review of the Signs and Symptoms
of Dementia and Brief Cognitive Tests Available in VA**
Evidence-based Synthesis Program

The second study drew consecutive, newly identified dementia patients (n=110) and controls matched on age and sex (n=138) from a primary care clinic.[66] This study compared the test performance using a cutoff of 29 with an age-adjusted cutoff score that raised the cutoff to 30 for ages 60-69, and lowered the cutoff by 1 point with each advancing age decade. Adjusting the cutoff score for age did not affect the sensitivity (86.4%), but improved the specificity of the STMS from 88.4% to 93.5%. To observe the effect of education without the confounding effects of dementia, the correlation of STMS total score with age and education was calculated within the control group only. The STMS appeared to be modestly influenced by age and education, with correlations of -0.34 (P = .0001) for age and 0.41 (P = .0001) for education. The study authors additionally noted that a severe language disturbance would preclude the use of the STMS.

KEY QUESTION #3. What are adverse consequences of using these measures?

Summary of findings

We found no evidence on adverse effects of the 6 cognitive tests of interest to VA. Three cross-sectional studies assessed the acceptability of dementia screening or diagnostic workup among older adults. The studies reported that high proportions of older adults were unwilling to be routinely tested for memory problems, or to undergo further diagnostic assessment for dementia after having positive results on cognitive screening tests. One survey determined that 80% of respondents wanted to know if they had dementia, but only 57% would agree to routine testing by a physician. Perceived harms included worry about losing insurance and fear of losing drivers license. The high refusal rates of screening and diagnostic workup indicate the need for further research to understand the psychological burden associated with cognitive tests and assessment for dementia.

Detailed description

The USPSTF 2003 review determined that most articles on the adverse effects of screening for dementia dealt primarily with genetic screening for increased risk of AD and the impact of disclosing the diagnosis of dementia.[74] Potential harms include psychological morbidity such as depressed mood, suicide, suicidal attempts and thoughts, and anxiety; as well as possible discrimination due to insurers and employers gaining access to screening results.[6, 74]

Our review found no literature on the adverse effects of the 6 cognitive tests of interest to VA. We found 2 studies that assessed the acceptability of dementia screening among older adults,[6,7] and 1 study that assessed refusal of diagnostic workup for dementia after screening.[8] Because the studies were cross-sectional surveys, we did not rate them for quality.

In 1 study, a mailed, self-administered questionnaire sent to residents of continuous care retirement communities (CCRCs) determined that the majority of respondents (51%) were not willing to be tested regularly for memory problems.[6] The questionnaire was sent to 500 residents aged 50 and older in two CCRCs in North Carolina, and excluded residents of assisted living and nursing homes, where the prevalence of diagnosed dementia would be greater. The survey contained 20 questions that addressed socio-demographic and health status, memory problems, depression, and medications; and also asked whether the respondent would like to be tested on a regular basis for memory problems and depression in 2 separate questions. Forty-nine percent of respondents were willing to be tested regularly for memory problems, and only 40% were interested in being screened regularly for depression. Acceptance of depression screening was highly correlated with acceptance of screening for memory problems: 97% of participants who were willing to accept routine depression screening would also accept routine screening for memory problems, whereas only 17% of those not willing to accept depression screening would accept routine memory screening. The study did not explore the reasons why residents were unwilling to be screened regularly for dementia, but the study investigators suggested that the high refusal rate indicates the need for further research to understand the psychological burden due to dementia screening, social stigmatization, health and long-term care insurance, employment discrimination, mistrust in the health care system in managing other medical conditions, institutionalization, and losing driving privileges.

In a screening and diagnosis study led by the same investigator, nearly half of patients with positive screening results refused diagnostic workup for dementia.[8] In this study, 3,340 patients aged 65 and older received cognitive screening, regardless of whether cognitive complaints were present, in 7 primary care practice centers in Indianapolis. Four hundred and thirty-four patients were eligible for diagnostic assessment, having made at least one error on a 6-item screening test[75] and subsequently scoring <=24 on a modified version of the Community Screening Instrument for Dementia.[76] Forty-eight percent of the patients with positive screening results refused further assessment for dementia. The proportion of refusals did not significantly differ between men (46.2%) and women (48.5%), or between African Americans (46.3%) and whites (50.4%), although the likelihood of refusal varied among age-race groups. Patients who made mistakes on orientation items were more willing to undergo the diagnostic assessment than those who did not make such mistakes. The study authors suggest that this finding may reflect the individual's perception as to whether or not s/he is likely to have the illness, in that patients who perceive themselves as asymptomatic may be less likely to desire to undergo a clinical evaluation.

A third study, published as an abstract,[7] sought to capture attitudes and perspectives toward dementia screening among 234 non-demented dwelling older adults (mean age 75) in North Carolina. This survey determined that 80% of respondents wanted to know if they had dementia, but only 57% would agree to routine testing by a physician. Perceived harms included worry about losing insurance (40%), and fear of losing drivers license (81%). Regression analysis determined that acceptance of routine dementia screening was associated with acceptance of routine screening for colon cancer (p<0.001), acceptance of routine depression screening (p<0.001), a belief that early detection improves treatment of dementia (p<0.001), and a fear that dementia leads to nursing home placement (p<0.038). The study investigators suggest that broad-based screening for early dementia may require targeted educational interventions regarding its benefits.

DISCUSSION

SIGNS AND SYMPTOMS OF DEMENTIA

Efforts to improve dementia case finding in general practice settings may be hampered by the protean manifestations of the disease, and the low sensitivity of many of the signs and symptoms encountered in practice. The utility of these signs and symptoms in effectively triaging patients for further diagnostic assessment would depend on the relative value placed on reducing false positive findings as compared to increasing dementia detection rates and reducing false negative rates. Determining the long-term benefits and harms of earlier and increased rates of dementia detection has been debated in the literature, but is largely beyond the scope of this review.

All of the signs and symptoms we evaluated were poorly sensitive in detecting mild dementia. This may reflect inter-individual variation in clinical manifestations of dementia, variations in the methods for detecting these signs and symptoms, or simply a reflection of the almost subclinical nature of early dementia.

The best studied of these symptoms are subjective memory complaints (SMC), which are theoretically attractive as a very brief initial assessment method in general practice settings. However, the presence of self-reported SMC does not correlate well with existing dementia. On the other hand, most cognitively intact persons do not have SMC, which may mean that in low prevalence settings, lack of SMC may be useful in identifying patients who could forego further dementia assessment. One potential consequence of routinely eliciting SMC in general practice patients is the likely high rate of false positives. If the finding of SMC would trigger further evaluation for dementia, this could lead to significant time pressures in general practice settings given that many of the "brief" assessment methods require 2 to 10 minutes to complete.

Of note, several large prospective cohort studies in different populations have found that elicited SMC are very common but of questionable significance, as they may not predict future cognitive decline.[77-79] Rather, studies have suggested self-reported SMC are associated with depression, anxiety, physical health and personality traits.[18, 45, 77]

Informant-reported memory complaints may better differentiate demented from non-demented individuals[18] and may be a promising area of inquiry for future case-finding approaches. The AD8 may be a promising very brief assessment instrument based partly on informant-reported memory complaints.[46] A number of additional studies have found that caregivers of demented patients are reliably able to assess their cognitive deficits.[45, 80-82] However, most of these studies have evaluated the use of longer questionnaires which may take some time to administer, and function almost as a proxy dementia screening tool.

Some neuropsychiatric symptoms such as apathy, hallucinations, and delusions are relatively uncommon in healthy elderly people and may suggest the need for further evaluation when present. Depression and anxiety, on the other hand, do not seem to be useful in distinguishing demented from non-demented individuals.

BRIEF MEASURES OF COGNITIVE FUNCTION AVAILABLE TO VA

The 6 measures available in VA all test for memory impairment, while apraxia and executive function (including a clock drawing test) are assessed in all measures except the BOMC. The assessment of other cognitive domains such as orientation, abstraction, and aphasia varies among the 6 measures (Table 5). A 2007 review by Holsinger, et al. discusses the cognitive domains in the DSM-IV criteria for dementia, and describes tasks used to assess each domain.[67]

Among the 6 tests, the Mini-Cog has the shortest administration time (2 to 4 minutes), and has been studied in a large population sample as well as in multi-ethnic samples. Sensitivity and specificity were high in 2 studies, while poor specificity in a third study may have resulted from inclusion of subjects with MCI.

The SLUMS examination had very high sensitivity and specificity in a VA population, and it allows for adjustment for education. However, the SLUMS has a longer administration time (approximately 7 minutes) compared with other tests, and has only been evaluated in 1 study.

The other 4 tests had various strengths and limitations. The STMS had high sensitivity and specificity in a primary care setting, but has been evaluated in only 2 studies. The GPCOG is unique in that it allows for the input of an informant; however, the specificity of the informant section by itself was low (49-66%). The BOMC was evaluated in a bi-racial population sample, and was found to misclassify more blacks than whites as impaired. Specificity varied widely among studies of the BOMC. The MoCA has the longest administration time among the 6 tests, and had low specificity (35-50%) in 2 of 3 studies.

LIMITATIONS

Our review does not address the relative value of various signs or symptoms in predicting future dementia. Also, because we excluded studies involving only patients with mild cognitive impairment (MCI) and because few included studies enrolled patients with very mild or very early dementia, these results may not be readily applicable to case-finding approaches designed to detect those patients with the earliest manifestations of disease.

The scope of this review was limited to the 6 brief cognitive measures identified as priorities for VA. There are many other cognitive measures available that are not covered in this review. Few studies have assessed the 6 instruments in VA populations, and though some of the study populations may be similar to VA populations, applicability to VA settings cannot be directly assumed. The adverse consequences of the 6 cognitive measures have not been studied.

FUTURE RESEARCH RECOMMENDATIONS

Consequences of expanded case-finding efforts

The utility and consequences of a targeted case-finding approach in VA primary care settings should be assessed. For instance, the utility of routinely asking about memory problems followed by a brief dementia assessment method in patients with a positive response should be studied. It would be critical in such a study to carefully assess both the rate and consequences of false-positive results, as well as the cost and time used to find one additional confirmed case of dementia.

The psychologic, financial, and quality of life consequences of both true- and false-positive dementia diagnoses should be more rigorously evaluated. High refusal rates of screening and diagnostic workup indicate the need for further research to understand the psychological burden associated with cognitive tests and assessment for dementia.

The role of caregivers in evaluating patients for dementia

The value of routinely asking patient caregivers about memory problems as an alternative to patient-reported memory complaints should be studied as well. Given a limited amount of literature suggesting informant characteristics may impact the reliability of informant report,[82] future studies of informant-administered instruments should also analyze the impact of the informant's relationship to the patient on the diagnostic utility of the instrument.

The reliability and validity of very brief informant assessment instruments such as the AD8 should be evaluated in different settings.

Evaluating combinations of signs and symptoms

Many of the signs and symptoms we examined were reported in isolation. Studies that examine the diagnostic utility of groups of signs and symptoms should be conducted.

Provider response to self-reported subjective memory complaints

Though the value of routine screening for dementia remains an active area of debate, subjective memory complaints are common enough that future studies, quality improvement, and education improvement efforts should ensure primary care providers are trained to feel comfortable having sensitive and holistic discussions with patients and their caregivers about memory loss. Studies should also address whether an assessment negative for dementia following a subjective memory complaint can be therapeutically useful.

Dementia and depression

Rates and consequences of the misclassification of dementia as depression (and vice versa) should be further studied.

Operating characteristics of the cognitive measures available in VA

The SLUMS and STMS tests have not been widely studied. Further studies are needed to assess the operating characteristics of these tests in various settings.

Of the 6 measures, only the BOMC and Mini-Cog have been evaluated in multi-ethnic samples. Further studies are needed to assess whether race or language biases affect the performance of the other cognitive measures.

Clinical utility of the cognitive measures available in VA

The perceived clinical utility of the GPCOG and Mini-Cog was examined in a narrative review and found to be equally high.[83] A similar survey among VA providers would be useful for determining preferences and utilities of the 6 measures available in VA. Because clinicians may need to use these assessment tools in busy primary care practices, studies should assess the instruments' ease of use, time to completion, and adverse effects in real-world VA settings.

REFERENCES

1.   Veterans Health Administration Office of the Assistant Deputy Under Secretary for Health for Policy and Planning. Projections of the prevalence and incidence of dementias including Alzheimer's Disease for the total, enrolled, and patient veteran populations aged 65 or over. 2004. *http://www4.va.gov/HEALTHPOLICYPLANNING/reports1.asp.*

2.   Yu W, Ravelo A, Wagner TH, et al. Prevalence and costs of chronic conditions in the VA health care system. *Med Care Res Rev.* Sep 2003;60(3 Suppl):146S-167S.

3.   U. S. Preventive Services Task Force. Screening for dementia: recommendations and rationale. *Am.* 91, 93, 95, 2003 Sep 2003;103(9):87.

4.   UK National Screening Committee. Policy on screening for Alzheimer's Disease. 26/03/09. *http://www.screening.nhs.uk/alzheimers.*

5.   Boustani M, Callahan CM, Unverzagt FW, et al. Implementing a screening and diagnosis program for dementia in primary care. *Journal of General Internal Medicine.* Jul 2005;20(7):572-577.

6.   Boustani M, Watson L, Fultz B, et al. Acceptance of dementia screening in continuous care retirement communities: a mailed survey. *Int J Geriatr Psychiatry.* Sep 2003;18(9):780-786.

7.   Hopkins JS, Watson LC, M. B, Perkins T, Fox C. What do healthy older adults think about dementia screening? *J Amer Geriatr Soc.* 2006;54:S189.

8.   Boustani M, Perkins AJ, Fox C, et al. Who refuses the diagnostic assessment for dementia in primary care? *Int J Geriatr Psychiatry.* Jun 2006;21(6):556-563.

9.   O'Connor DW, Pollitt PA, Hyde JB, Brook CP, Reiss BB, Roth M. Do general practitioners miss dementia in elderly patients? *Bmj.* Oct 29 1988;297(6656):1107-1110.

10.   Sternberg SA, Wolfson C, Baumgarten M. Undetected dementia in community-dwelling older people: the Canadian Study of Health and Aging. *J Am Geriatr Soc.* Nov 2000;48(11):1430-1434.

11.   Valcour VG, Masaki KH, Curb JD, Blanchette PL. The detection of dementia in the primary care setting. *Arch Intern Med.* Oct 23 2000;160(19):2964-2968.

12.   National Chronic Care Consortium and the Alzheimer's Association. Tools for early identification, assessment, and treatment for people with Alzheimer's disease and dementia. 1998, revised June 2003. *A publication of the Chronic Care Networks for Alzheimer's Disease Initiative. Available at www.alz.org/national/documents/ccn-ad03.pdf.*

13.   Whiting P, Rutjes AW, Reitsma JB, et al. The development of QUADAS: a tool for the quality assessment of studies of diagnostic accuracy included in systematic reviews. *BMC Med Res Methodol.* Nov 10 2003;3:25.

14. Whiting P, Harbord R, Kleijnen J, Whiting P, Harbord R, Kleijnen J. No role for quality scores in systematic reviews of diagnostic accuracy studies. *BMC Med Res Methodol.* 2005;5:19.

15. Mitchell AJ. The clinical significance of subjective memory complaints in the diagnosis of mild cognitive impairment and dementia: a meta-analysis. *Int J Geriatr Psychiatry.* Nov 2008;23(11):1191-1202.

16. Lavery LL, Lu SY, Chang CC, Saxton J, Ganguli M. Cognitive assessment of older primary care patients with and without memory complaints. *J Gen Intern Med.* Jul 2007;22(7):949-954.

17. Ganguli M, Du Y, Rodriguez EG, et al. Discrepancies in information provided to primary care physicians by patients with and without dementia: the Steel Valley Seniors Survey. *Am J Geriatr Psychiatry.* May 2006;14(5):446-455.

18. Carr DB, Gray S, Baty J, Morris JC. The value of informant versus individual's complaints of memory impairment in early dementia. *Neurology.* Dec 12 2000;55(11):1724-1726.

19. Tatsch MF, Bottino CM, Azevedo D, et al. Neuropsychiatric symptoms in Alzheimer disease and cognitively impaired, nondemented elderly from a community-based sample in Brazil: prevalence and relationship with dementia severity. *Am J Geriatr Psychiatry.* May 2006;14(5):438-445.

20. Lyketsos CG, Lopez O, Jones B, Fitzpatrick AL, Breitner J, DeKosky S. Prevalence of neuropsychiatric symptoms in dementia and mild cognitive impairment: results from the cardiovascular health study. *Jama.* Sep 25 2002;288(12):1475-1483.

21. Lyketsos CG, Steinberg M, Tschanz JT, Norton MC, Steffens DC, Breitner JC. Mental and behavioral disturbances in dementia: findings from the Cache County Study on Memory in Aging. *Am J Psychiatry.* May 2000;157(5):708-714.

22. Lopponen M, Raiha I, Isoaho R, Vahlberg T, Kivela SL. Diagnosing cognitive impairment and dementia in primary health care -- a more active approach is needed. *Age Ageing.* Nov 2003;32(6):606-612.

23. Lazarus LW, Newton N, Cohler B, Lesser J, Schweon C. Frequency and presentation of depressive symptoms in patients with primary degenerative dementia. *Am J Psychiatry.* Jan 1987;144(1):41-45.

24. Hancock P, Larner AJ. Diagnostic utility of the Pittsburgh sleep Quality Index in memory clinics. *Int J Geriatr Psychiatry.* Mar 31 2009.

25. Tractenberg RE, Singer CM, Kaye JA. Symptoms of sleep disturbance in persons with Alzheimer's disease and normal elderly. *J Sleep Res.* Jun 2005;14(2):177-185.

26.   Giron MS, Forsell Y, Bernsten C, Thorslund M, Winblad B, Fastbom J. Sleep problems in a very old population: drug use and clinical correlates. *J Gerontol A Biol Sci Med Sci.* Apr 2002;57(4):M236-240.

27.   Marion MH, Qurashi M, Marshall G, Foster O. Is REM sleep behaviour disorder (RBD) a risk factor of dementia in idiopathic Parkinson's disease? *J Neurol.* Feb 2008;255(2):192-196.

28.   Allan LM, Ballard CG, Burn DJ, Kenny RA. Prevalence and severity of gait disorders in Alzheimer's and non-Alzheimer's dementias. *J Am Geriatr Soc.* Oct 2005;53(10):1681-1687.

29.   O'Keeffe ST, Kazeem H, Philpott RM. Gait disturbance in Alzheimer's disease: A clinical study. *Age Ageing.* 1996;25:313-316.

30.   Waite LM, Broe GA, Creasey H, Grayson D, Edelbrock D, O'Toole B. Neurological signs, aging, and the neurodegenerative syndromes. *Arch Neurol.* Jun 1996;53(6):498-502.

31.   Huff FJ, Boller F, Lucchelli F, Querriera R, Beyer J, Belle S. The neurologic examination in patients with probable Alzheimer's disease. *Arch Neurol.* Sep 1987;44(9):929-932.

32.   Lee AY, Jeong SH, Choi BH, Sohn EH, Chui H. Pulse pressure correlates with leukoaraiosis in Alzheimer disease. *Arch Gerontol Geriatr.* Mar-Apr 2006;42(2):157-166.

33.   Brown LB, Ott BR, Papandonatos GD, Sui Y, Ready RE, Morris JC. Prediction of on-road driving performance in patients with early Alzheimer's disease. *J Am Geriatr Soc.* Jan 2005;53(1):94-98.

34.   Jonker C, Geerlings MI, Schmand B. Are memory complaints predictive for dementia? A review of clinical and population-based studies. *Int J Geriatr Psychiatry.* Nov 2000;15(11):983-991.

35.   Jungwirth S, Fischer P, Weissgram S, Kirchmeyr W, Bauer P, Tragl KH. Subjective memory complaints and objective memory impairment in the Vienna-Transdanube aging community. *J Am Geriatr Soc.* Feb 2004;52(2):263-268.

36.   Tobiansky R, Blizard R, Livingston G, Mann A. The Gospel Oak Study stage IV: the clinical relevance of subjective memory impairment in older people. *Psychol Med.* Jul 1995;25(4):779-786.

37.   St John P, Montgomery P, St John P, Montgomery P. Is subjective memory loss correlated with MMSE scores or dementia? *J Geriatr Psychiatry Neurol.* Jun 2003;16(2):80-83.

38.   Jungwirth S, Weissgram S, Zehetmayer S, Tragl KH, Fischer P. VITA: subtypes of mild cognitive impairment in a community-based cohort at the age of 75 years. *Int J Geriatr Psychiatry.* May 2005;20(5):452-458.

39. Lam LC, Lui VW, Tam CW, et al. Subjective memory complaints in Chinese subjects with mild cognitive impairment and early Alzheimer's disease. *Int J Geriatr Psychiatry.* Sep 2005;20(9):876-882.

40. Chong MS, Chin JJ, Saw SM, et al. Screening for dementia in the older Chinese with a single question test on progressive forgetfulness. *Int J Geriatr Psychiatry.* May 2006;21(5):442-448.

41. Grut M, Jorm AF, Fratiglioni L, Forsell Y, Viitanen M, Winblad B. Memory complaints of elderly people in a population survey: variation according to dementia stage and depression. *J Am Geriatr Soc.* Dec 1993;41(12):1295-1300.

42. Purser JL, Fillenbaum GG, Wallace RB, Purser JL, Fillenbaum GG, Wallace RB. Memory complaint is not necessary for diagnosis of mild cognitive impairment and does not predict 10-year trajectories of functional disability, word recall, or short portable mental status questionnaire limitations. *J Am Geriatr Soc.* Feb 2006;54(2):335-338.

43. Crooks VC, Buckwalter JG, Petitti DB, Brody KK, Yep RL. Self-reported severe memory problems as a screen for cognitive impairment and dementia. *Dementia.* 2005;4(4):539-551.

44. Tierney MC, Szalai JP, Snow WG, Fisher RH. The prediction of Alzheimer disease. The role of patient and informant perceptions of cognitive deficits. *Arch Neurol.* May 1996;53(5):423-427.

45. McGlone J, Gupta S, Humphrey D, Oppenheimer S, Mirsen T, Evans DR. Screening for early dementia using memory complaints from patients and relatives. *Arch Neurol.* Nov 1990;47(11):1189-1193.

46. Galvin JE, Roe CM, Xiong C, et al. Validity and reliability of the AD8 informant interview in dementia. *Neurology.* Dec 12 2006;67(11):1942-1948.

47. Galvin JE, Roe CM, Coats MA, et al. Patient's rating of cognitive ability: using the AD8, a brief informant interview, as a self-rating tool to detect dementia. *Arch Neurol.* May 2007;64(5):725-730.

48. Cummings JL, Mega M, Gray K, Rosenberg-Thompson S, Carusi DA, Gornbein J. The Neuropsychiatric Inventory: comprehensive assessment of psychopathology in dementia. *Neurology.* Dec 1994;44(12):2308-2314.

49. McKhann G, Drachman D, Folstein M, Katzman R, Price D, Stadlan EM. Clinical diagnosis of Alzheimer's disease: report of the NINCDS-ADRDA Work Group under the auspices of Department of Health and Human Services Task Force on Alzheimer's Disease. *Neurology.* Jul 1984;34(7):939-944.

50. Katzman R, Brown T, Fuld P, Peck A, Schechter R, Schimmel H. Validation of a short Orientation-Memory-Concentration Test of cognitive impairment. *Am J Psychiatry.* Jun 1983;140(6):734-739.

51.   Boustani M, Peterson B, Hanson L, et al. Screening for dementia in primary care: a summary of the evidence for the U.S. Preventive Services Task Force. *Ann Intern Med.* Jun 3 2003;138(11):927-937.

52.   Fillenbaum G, Heyman A, Williams K, Prosnitz B, Burchett B. Sensitivity and specificity of standardized screens of cognitive impairment and dementia among elderly black and white community residents. *J Clin Epidemiol.* 1990;43(7):651-660.

53.   Stuss DT, Meiran N, Guzman DA, Lafleche G, Willmer J. Do long tests yield a more accurate diagnosis of dementia than short tests? A comparison of 5 neuropsychological tests. *Arch Neurol.* Oct 1996;53(10):1033-1039.

54.   Davous P, Lamour Y, Debrand E, Rondot P. A comparative evaluation of the short orientation memory concentration test of cognitive impairment. *J Neurol Neurosurg Psychiatry.* Oct 1987;50(10):1312-1317.

55.   Costa PT, Jr., Williams TF, Somerfield MR, Albert MS, Nutters NM, Folstein MF, et al. *Recognition and Initial Assessment of Alzheimer's Disease and Related Dementias. Clinical Practice Guideline no. 19.* Rockville, MD: U.S. Department of Health and Human Services, Public Health Service, Agency for Health Care Policy and Research AHCPR Publication no. 97-0702; 1996.

56.   Brodaty H, Pond D, Kemp NM, et al. The GPCOG: a new screening test for dementia designed for general practice. *J Am Geriatr Soc.* Mar 2002;50(3):530-534.

57.   Basic D, Khoo A, Conforti D, et al. Rowland Universal Dementia Assessment Scale, Mini-Mental State Examination and General Practitioner Assessment of Cognition in a multicultural cohort of community-dwelling older persons with early dementia. *Australian Psychologist.* 2009;44(1):40-53.

58.   Borson S, Scanlan JM, Chen P, Ganguli M. The Mini-Cog as a screen for dementia: validation in a population-based sample. *J Am Geriatr Soc.* Oct 2003;51(10):1451-1454.

59.   Borson S, Scanlan JM, Watanabe J, Tu SP, Lessig M. Simplifying detection of cognitive impairment: comparison of the Mini-Cog and Mini-Mental State Examination in a multi-ethnic sample. *J Am Geriatr Soc.* May 2005;53(5):871-874.

60.   Kaufer DI, Williams CS, Braaten AJ, Gill K, Zimmerman S, Sloane PD. Cognitive screening for dementia and mild cognitive impairment in assisted living: comparison of 3 tests. *J Am Med Dir Assoc.* Oct 2008;9(8):586-593.

61.   Smith T, Gildeh N, Holmes C. The Montreal Cognitive Assessment: validity and utility in a memory clinic setting. *Can J Psychiatry.* May 2007;52(5):329-332.

62.   Luis CA, Keegan AP, Mullan M. Cross validation of the Montreal Cognitive Assessment in community dwelling older adults residing in the Southeastern US. *Int J Geriatr Psychiatry.* 2009;24(2):197-201.

63.   Nasreddine ZS, Phillips NA, Bedirian V, et al. The Montreal Cognitive Assessment, MoCA: a brief screening tool for mild cognitive impairment. *J Am Geriatr Soc.* Apr 2005;53(4):695-699.

64.   Tariq SH, Tumosa N, Chibnall JT, Perry MH, 3rd, Morley JE. Comparison of the Saint Louis University mental status examination and the mini-mental state examination for detecting dementia and mild neurocognitive disorder--a pilot study. *Am J Geriatr Psychiatry.* Nov 2006;14(11):900-910.

65.   Kokmen E, Naessens JM, Offord KP. A short test of mental status: description and preliminary results. *Mayo Clin Proc.* Apr 1987;62(4):281-288.

66.   Kokmen E, Smith GE, Petersen RC, Tangalos E, et al. The Short Test of Mental Status: Correlations with standardized psychometric testing. *Arch Neurol.* Jul 1991;48(7):725-728.

67.   Holsinger T, Deveau J, Boustani M, Williams JW, Jr. Does this patient have dementia? *Jama.* Jun 6 2007;297(21):2391-2404.

68.   Borson S, Scanlan J, Brush M, Vitaliano P, Dokmak A. The mini-cog: a cognitive 'vital signs' measure for dementia screening in multi-lingual elderly. *Int J Geriatr Psychiatry.* Nov 2000;15(11):1021-1027.

69.   Blessed G, Tomlinson BE, Roth M. The association between quantitative measures of dementia and of senile change in the cerebral grey matter of elderly subjects. *Br J Psychiatry.* Jul 1968;114(512):797-811.

70.   Froehlich TE, Bogardus ST, Jr., Inouye SK. Dementia and race: are there differences between African Americans and Caucasians? *J Am Geriatr Soc.* Apr 2001;49(4):477-484.

71.   Lourenco RA, Filho Ribeiro ST. The accuracy of the Mini-Cog in screening low-educated elderly for dementia. *J Am Geriatr Soc.* Feb 2006;54(2):376-377; author reply 377-378.

72.   Borson S, Scanlan JM. Response to Drs. Lourenco and Ribeiro Filho. *J Am Geriatr Soc.* Feb 2006;54(2):377-378.

73.   Nasreddine Z. The Montreal Cognitive Assessment - MoCA. *http://www.mocatest.org/ Accessed Feb 1, 2010.*

74.   Boustani M, Peterson B, Hanson L. Screening for dementia. Systematic evidence review. *U.S. Preventive Services Task Force. Agency for Healthcare Research and Quality, Rockville, MD. http://www.ahrq.gov/clinic/uspstf/uspsdeme.htm* 2003.

75.   Callahan CM, Unverzagt FW, Hui SL, et al. Six-item screener to identify cognitive impairment among potential subjects for clinical research. *Medical Care.* Sep 2002;40(9):771-781.

76.   Hall KS, Hendrie HC, Brittain HM, et al. The development of a dementia screening interview in two distinct languages. *Int J Meth Psychiatric Res.* 1993;3:1-28.

77. Comijs HC, Deeg DJH, Dik MG, Twisk JWR, Jonker C. Memory complaints; the association with psycho-affective and health problems and the role of personality characteristics: A 6-year follow-up study. *J Affect Disord.* 2002;72(2):157-165.

78. Park MH, Min JY, Min HY, Lee HJ, Lee DH, Song MS. Subjective memory complaints and clinical characteristics in elderly Koreans: A questionnaire survey. *International Journal of Nursing Studies.* 2007;44(8):1400-1405.

79. Blazer DG, Hays JC, Fillenbaum GG, Gold DT. Memory complaint as a predictor of cognitive decline: a comparison of African American and White elders. *J Aging Health.* May 1997;9(2):171-184.

80. Jorm AF. Methods of screening for dementia: a meta-analysis of studies comparing an informant questionnaire with a brief cognitive test. *Alzheimer Dis Assoc Disord.* Sep 1997;11(3):158-162.

81. Koss E, Patterson MB, Ownby R, Stuckey JC, Whitehouse PJ. Memory evaluation in Alzheimer's disease. Caregivers' appraisals and objective testing. *Arch Neurol.* Jan 1993;50(1):92-97.

82. Shen J, Gao S, Unverzagt FW, et al. Validation analysis of informant's ratings of cognitive function in African Americans and Nigerians. *Int J Geriatr Psychiatry.* Jul 2006;21(7):618-625.

83. Milne A, Culverwell A, Guss R, Tuppen J, Whelton R. Screening for dementia in primary care: a review of the use, efficacy and quality of measures. *Int Psychogeriatr.* Oct 2008;20(5):911-926.

APPENDIX A. SEARCH STRATEGY

Symbol	Concept	Search Strategy (PubMed)
D	Dementia	"dementia"[MeSH Terms] OR "dementia"[All Fields]
SS	Signs + Symptoms	((((("signs + symptoms"[MeSH Terms] OR ("signs"[All Fields] + "symptoms"[All Fields]) OR "signs + symptoms"[All Fields]) OR (warning sign[All Fields] OR warning signal[All Fields] OR warning signal/precue[All Fields] OR warning signals[All Fields] OR warning signs[All Fields] OR warning signs/symptoms[All Fields])) OR (red flag[All Fields] OR red flagging[All Fields] OR red flags[All Fields])) OR presenting[All Fields]) OR (suspect[All Fields] OR suspected[All Fields])) OR (predict[All Fields] OR predictor[All Fields] OR predictors[All Fields])
CS	Cross-Sectional Studies	"Cross-Sectional Studies"[Mesh]
SR	Systematic Review Subset	systematic[sb]
G	Guidelines, Consensus Statement Publication Type	Guideline [pt] OR Consensus Development Conference [pt]
T	Specific Tests	(("montreal cognitive assessment"[tiab]))) OR (("moca"[tiab]))) OR (("slums"[tiab]))) OR (("st louis university mental status"[tiab]))) OR (("saint louis university mental status"[tiab]))) OR (("short test of mental status"[tiab]))) OR (("STMS"[tiab]))) OR (("General Practitioner Assessment of Cognition"[tiab]))) OR (("GPCog"[tiab]))) OR (("mini-cog"[tiab]))) OR (("mini cog"[tiab]))) OR (("orientation memory concentration"[tiab]))) OR (("bomc"[tiab])))) NOT ((poverty areas[mesh]))

All searches were performed in July of 2009

Dementia Review #1 Key Question #1
PubMed
Primary Studies
(D + SS + CS) = 518
Secondary Studies (systematic reviews, guidelines or consensus statements only not general reviews)
((D + SS) + (SR OR G)) = 322

Additional databases

Cochrane central register of controlled trials and database of abstracts of reviews of effects

1	dementia.mp.
2	(signs and symptoms).mp
3	warning sign.mp.
4	warning signal.mp.
5	red flag*.mp.
6	presenting.mp.
7	suspect.mp.
8	suspected.mp.
9	predict*.mp
10	8 or 6 or 4 or 3 or 7 or 9 or 2 or 5
11	1 and 10

229 results after de-duplication 201

CINAHL

S1	("dementia") or (MH "Dementia+")
S2	("signs and symptoms") or (MH "Signs and Symptoms (Non-Cinahl)")
S3	"warning signs"
S4	"warning signal"
S5	"red flag*"
S6	"presenting"
S7	"suspect"
S8	"suspected"
S9	"predict"
S10	predictor*
S11	S2 or S3 or S4 or S5 or S6 or S7 or S8 or S9 or S10
S12	("dementia") or (MM "Dementia+")
S13	S11 and S12
S14	S11 and S12 Narrow by Subject: Major Heading0: - Dementia

367 results after de-duplication 309

PsychINFO

1	exp *Dementia/	30642
2	(signs and symptoms).mp. [mp=title, abstract, heading word, table of contents, key concepts]	5567
3	warning sign.mp. or exp Warnings/	738

4   red flag.mp.   42
5   red flags.mp.   77
6   exp Symptoms/ or presenting.mp.   131298
7   suspect.mp.   1854
8   suspected.mp. 4720
9   predict.mp.   36261
10   predictor.mp.   27521
11   predictors.mp.   38646
12   6 or 11 or 3 or 7 or 9 or 2 or 8 or 4 or 10 or 5   222250
13   1 and 12   4251
14   limit 13 to ("0800 literature review" or "0830 systematic review" or 1200 meta analysis)

208 Results after de-duplication 192

AGELINE

Title: dementia
AND
Title: "signs and symptoms" ; "warning sign" ; "warning signal" ; "red flag" ; "red flags" ;
presenting ; suspect ; suspected ; predict ; predictor

39 items after de-duplication 30 unique

We also re-executed the search described in Mitchell, 2008 in Medline.

(subjective memory OR memory complaint* OR memory difficult* [abstract]) AND (Dementia
OR Alzheimer* OR mild cognitive [abstract]) AND (validity OR diagnosis OR sensitivity OR
specificity OR accuracy OR re receiveOperator OR ROC [full text]) limited to 2008-Sept 2009
(date of search)

79 Results

Dementia Review #1 Key Question #2 & 3

PubMed
(D + T) = 54

Additional databases (named tests were searched in the following databases)
Cochrane central register of controlled trials and database of abstracts of reviews of effects: 27
Results, after de-duplication 0
HAPI: 24 Results, after de-duplication 23
PsycINFO: 87 Results, after de-duplication 74
CINAHL: 48 Results, after de-duplication 44

APPENDIX B. INCLUSION/EXCLUSION CRITERIA

Author, Year_____   Title or ID#_____

	Key words or categories:

1. Do any of the following constitute the study population:
   a. A community sample of persons age 60+ that includes non-demented
      individuals as well as patients with mild to moderate dementia ....❑
   b. Patients with newly diagnosed, mild to moderate dementia ....❑
   c. Non-demented individuals aged 60+...❑
   d. None of the above..STOP
 	
2. Does the study use a standard criterion for diagnosing dementia?
   a. No ....STOP
   b. Yes (e.g. DSM-IV)..❑	

3. Does the study evaluate any of the following cognitive tests:
   Blessed Orientation-Memory-Concentration Test (BOMC) ....❑
   Mini-Cog ....❑
   General Practitioner Assessment of Cognition (GPCOG)............................❑
   Short Test of Mental Status (STMS) ....❑
   St. Louis University Mental Status Exam (SLUMS) ....❑
   Montreal Cognitive Assessment (MoCA) ....❑
   None of the above...proceed to Q4
 	
4. Does the study provide prevalence or other descriptive data on signs and/or
   symptoms of dementia?*
   a. No ....STOP
   b. Yes ....❑
 	
5. Is the text of the article in English?
   a. No ....STOP
   b. Yes ....❑
 	
6. If this article meets no other criterion, should it be saved for background or
   discussion?
   a. No ....STOP
   b. Yes: clinical guidelines...❑
   c. Yes: narrative review with potentially useful references............................❑
   d. Yes: qualitative study discussing relevant signs and symptoms.................❑
   e. Yes: other, specify..❑
	Notes

Circle the Key Question(s) to which this article applies:

   1. What signs and symptoms should prompt VA providers to assess cognitive function as part of an initial diagnostic workup for dementia?

   2. Which measures of cognitive function provide the optimal sensitivity, specificity, and time to administer, and are readily available within the VA?

   3. What are adverse consequences of using these measures?

* Examples of data that do not meet criteria for item 4 include epidemiologic risk factors for dementia; diagnostic imaging, laboratory, or physiological tests (e.g. sense of smell; cerebrospinal fluid studies; indicators of acute confusion; predictors of DNR orders

APPENDIX C.   QUADAS CRITERIA FOR EVALUATING DIAGNOSTIC ACCURACY STUDIES

Table 2: The Quadas tool

Item		Yes	No	Unclear
1.	Was the spectrum of patients representative of the patients who will receive the test in practice?	( )	( )	( )
2.	Were selection criteria clearly described?	( )	( )	( )
3.	Is the reference standard likely to correctly classify the target condition?	( )	( )	( )
4.	Is the time period between reference standard and index test short enough to be reasonably sure that the target condition did not change between the two tests?	( )	( )	( )
5.	Did the whole sample or a random selection of the sample, receive verification using a reference standard of diagnosis?	( )	( )	( )
6.	Did patients receive the same reference standard regardless of the index test result?	( )	( )	( )
7.	Was the reference standard independent of the index test (i.e. the index test did not form part of the reference standard)?	( )	( )	( )
8.	Was the execution of the index test described in sufficient detail to permit replication of the test?	( )	( )	( )
9.	Was the execution of the reference standard described in sufficient detail to permit its replication?	( )	( )	( )
10.	Were the index test results interpreted without knowledge of the results of the reference standard?	( )	( )	( )
11.	Were the reference standard results interpreted without knowledge of the results of the index test?	( )	( )	( )
12.	Were the same clinical data available when test results were interpreted as would be available when the test is used in practice?	( )	( )	( )
13.	Were uninterpretable/ intermediate test results reported?	( )	( )	( )
14.	Were withdrawals from the study explained?	( )	( )	( )

Source: Whiting P, Rutjes AW, Reitsma JB, Bossuyt PM, Kleijnen J, Whiting P, et al. The development of QUADAS: a tool for the quality assessment of studies of diagnostic accuracy included in systematic reviews. BMC Medical Research Methodology 2003;3:25. Used with permission.

APPENDIX D. PEER REVIEW COMMENTS

Reviewer	Comment	Response
Question 1. Are the objectives, scope, and methods for this review clearly described?		
1	Yes. Objective scope and methods are clearly described. The report is very succinct and to the point. However, I did not see QUADAS criteria fully explained. This should be explicitly described so a reader can independently evaluate how you did your evaluation.	Noted. We have clarified in the Methods that the details of the QUADAS criteria are listed in Appendix C.
2	Yes. Would be very helpful to have a glossary of terms to help non-expert readers (e.g., many policy-makers) understand the statistical terms (e.g., sensitivity, specificity, prevalence, incidence, positive/negative predictive value, screening, etc.) and other technical terms (e.g., stereognosis and graphesthesia). It is important that the methods, results, and discussion/conclusions/recommendations be clear in layperson as well as technical terms.	Will include glossary and we've tried to modify the language.
3	Yes. (No comment)	Noted.
4	Yes. Did you consider examining warning signs in combination rather than singly (e.g., memory complaint in combination with behavioral symptom such as apathy or driving violation). This may improve the discriminative properties of the warning signs. If you have not considered this – would you consider examining these warning signs in combination? That is a likely scenario for clinical use. It is unclear to me the extent to which you considered studies that discussed informants identification of (sic)	We've actually added some studies and narrative re: informant report. We added the suggestion re: consideration of examining these warning signs in combination to our future studies section.
5	Yes. I believe that this review sheds light on important questions and is very clear in the way it answers these questions with evidence based response/discussion. I found it to be very informative in looking at a large body of literature to answer specific questions that are very clinically relevant in dementia diagnosis/ recognition.	Noted.
Question 2. Is there any indication of bias in our synthesis of the evidence?		
1	There is no evident bias in synthesis of evidence however, limiting to just studies of persons with dementia severely limits the applicability of this review to the world that we work in. In general there is too much emphasis on diagnosis when this is an imperfect process at best. There are individuals with severe levels of MCI or MCI-R, for example, who suffer in multiple ways due to their disability. We need to identify these patients (Veterans) and "treat" them as well and often we do not address impairment until it is severe enough to be able to classify as "probable dementia."	The scope of this review was limited to dementia. However, we agree that Veterans with cognitive impairment non-dementia (CIND) are an important patient population. The best practices for assessment and management of patients with CIND may warrant a separate evidence review.
2	No.	Noted.

Reviewer	Comment	Response
3	Yes. Not a systematic bias but an odd ignoring of certain literature with over emphasis on other papers.	Noted. We have responded to the specific points raised in Question 4.
4	No - However, some who are strong advocates for screening might complain that you have only looked for adverse effects of screening, and have not considered adverse effects of missed diagnosis (e.g., worsened chronic disease control). To my knowledge these studies have not been done, so I personally do not believe this is a strong criticism.	Although identifying the consequences of falsely negative results from brief mental status tests was not within the scope of Key Question 2, we agree that the effects of case-finding and missed diagnoses on the improvement or worsening of patient outcomes are important considerations.
5	No bias was visible in this review.	Noted.
Question 3. *Are there any studies on dementia signs and symptoms, or on the cognitive measures of interest to the VA, that we have overlooked?*		
1	Yes. My only concern here is again the filter that was used, as a general concern about the completeness of your literature search. Some studies have used tools that estimate a high probability of dementia based on prior validation studies with that instrument. You need to be careful to include studies that also have this approximation even if subjects were not even ostensibly diagnosed. You did this when including Crooks' study, a study I know well and these patients were not "diagnosed" but had an approximation of diagnosis applied. I conducted a study of memory impairment in Veterans and concern about impairment as a strong predictor where there was a high probability of dementia that was dictated by conservative cut-points from prior validation research. This should have been considered for inclusion (perhaps it was) especially because it was done within the VA.	This was designed to be a review case-finding tools rather than tools that are predictive of future dementia. Re: the Crooks paper - we did not include this as a primary study - it was included as part of the Mitchell review and we did, in our revisions, clarify the weaknesses of individual studies from the Mitchell review including Crooks (we agree they did not use a gold standard for dementia assessment).
2	None that I'm aware of specifically.	Noted.
3	Yes. I think you gloss over a sizable literature on informant reported memory problems in favor of focusing on a patient's own subjective complaints. It has been suggested repeatedly that subjective memory complaints on the part of the patient are frequently associated with anxiety and depression while the reports of informants (and a literature suggesting that spouses are the best informants) are more related to actual cognitive decline yet you avoid discussion of the problems with an individual's complaints and ignore informant complaints almost completely. The MMSE has many problems and is just about as insensitive as the mini-Cog and short Blessed (BOMC), but it has the largest body of literature by far and is most familiar to actual providers.	We've added some more discussion points about informant reported memory problems. We had not included some studies (eg - Archer 2007) because they fell outside inclusion criteria (assessing MCI in this case). Many studies investigate association with future cognitive decline. However, we agree it is important to clarify some of the potential weaknesses of patient reported complaints and acknowledge the potential role of informant report. We've added the Jorm 1997 review to our dicussion, though it really looks at the value of longer informant questionnaires which is slightly different from "signs/sx" (which a very brief elicitation of SMC might approximate). We added Carr 2000 as well. Re: MMSE - it was simply outside of our review's scope - the scope of our report reflects the Dementia Steering Committee's interests - they were interested in literature about six commonly used alternatives to MMSE.

Reviewer	Comment	Response
4	See comment above concerning dementia warning signs considered in combination, rather than in isolation. Also – there are other warning signs type instruments – see for example: Galvin JE, et al, The AD8, a brief informant interview to detect dementia,Neurology 2005;65:559-564. See also the following article that may help to illuminate the role of informant information and its usefulness in guiding diagnosis of dementia. Informant ratings of cognitive decline in old age: validation against change on cognitive tests over 7 to 8 years. Jorm AF. Christensen H. Korten AE. Jacomb PA. Henderson AS. Psychological Medicine. 30(4):981-5, 2000 Jul. Validation analysis of informant's ratings of cognitive function in African Americans and Nigerians. Shen J. Gao S. Unverzagt FW. Ogunniyi A. Baiyewu O. Gureje O. Hendrie HC. Hall KS. International Journal of Geriatric Psychiatry. 21(7):618-25, 2006 Jul.	Agree - we've added more information re: informant report including the articles you mention and others we found. We mentioned the Shen study in the discussion and future studies section. The warning signs in combination is an interesting point and has not been well-studied - we've added it to suggestions for future studies.
5	Yes. One important document to consider (if not already considered) is the Alzheimer's association 10 warning signs for dementia. I find that these warning signs, which were recently updated after significant input, are worth sincere evaluation as dementia warning signs.	The suggested document was included in the draft report.
Question 4. Please write additional suggestions or comments below: If applicable, please indicate the page and line numbers from the draft report.		
1	I am concerned about restrictive (and traditional) intentions of this work: 1) find ways to identify and diagnose dementia patients or those at high risk; 2) do this in a brief "cost-effective" way; and 3) find signs and symptoms because screening poses too much of a burden. Medical providers are drilled on signs and symptoms of CHF, for example, and we have Review of System questions to identify potential risk. Practitioners are often uncomfortable about screening or ruling in or out dementia. Your review suggests that warning signs are not helpful – at least there is little evidence thus far. Perhaps more attention needs to be put on how to teach providers how to sensitively and comfortably discuss cognitive concerns. Your review and others like it suggest that memory complaints might not predict dementia (though I believe that my study did predict it) and therefore they do not need to be addressed. I think you should include a discussion about addressing patient complaints regarding memory because of the inherent need to do that as an effective and sensitive practitioner regardless of the underlying reason for the complaint. A normal screen can be very reassuring and may address significant anxiety. With all that said, this is a very professional, well organized and thoughtful review. This has real value to VA and its Veterans.	These are well-considered and well-put concerns. Much of this debate is beyond the scope of this review. Because the issue of screening for dementia (as distinguished from case-finding) has been widely debated and there are already excellent publications and reviews outlining both sides of this debate, we have tried to make clear this review does not address the relative value of widespread screening for dementia. The points re: training providers how to sensitively and comprehensively address memory concerns, and the reassurance that a normal screen can offer a patient are well-taken. We have inserted some suggested future areas of study along these lines.

Reviewer	Comment	Response
2	Please see attached document with comments in Track Changes. This is an important, well-written report. But we need the methods/results/discussion/ conclusions/ clearly presented in non-technical terms so that non-expert policy-makers will understand the recommendations for further action. Don't "hide" the results and recommendations within technical terms.	Noted, and we've modified the language.
2	Background in body and Exec Summary, Lines 3-7: these data come from VA Allocation Resource Center (ARC) data, which are on the VA Intranet only and are not public. Citation 1 references the ARC website on the VA Intranet. It has not yet been decided what parts of the DSC Report can be made public. An alternative would be to quote the 2004 VA dementia projection from the VHA Office of the Assistant Deputy Under Secretary for Health for Policy and Planning, also posted on the internet at www1.va.gov/vhareorg/reports.htm. There is also a 2003 publication by VA HERC that gives some dementia cost data from 1999 (Yu W, et al, 2003). These public data are mentioned on p. 1-2 of the DSC report.	We have replaced this paragraph using data from the suggested references.
2	Page v line 27; also page 17 line 12: sterognosis and graphesthesia: use layperson terms in addition to the technical terms, for non-expert readers	We have defined these terms in the text, and added them to the Glossary.
2	Methods, page 3, line 8: citation 13 is an internal memo, I'm not sure it is appropriate to cite it here.	We agree and have deleted reference 13.
2	Page 4, lines 5-6: Can you say more about the decision to exclude studies on signs and symptoms that predict future incident dementia? (e-mail discussion copied here) ...A little more explicit would be great. If you could amplify in the report just a bit, like your sentence below that I highlighted in yellow, that would be helpful. It may be just a matter of adding the "layperson" wording, or repeating it in the Study Selection section as you did in the Background section.	This was really designed as a review of case-finding tools rather than a review of tools that are predictive of future dementia. Our review does not address the latter issue and I hope this is clear to the reading audience. Given the lack of convincing evidence re: screening for dementia and the lack of clear consensus around this issue, we had thought that a review of methods for predicting dementia would be less applicable. We tried to frame this issue in the introduction, but again please let me know if we should be more explicit.
2	Page 16, line 9: Word(s) missing? Check sentence: "...questionnaires were completed (not?) by caregivers of demented participants, but by the non-demented participants themselves (22)."	We have clarified this sentence to read as follows: "Results from the third study are more difficult to interpret because sleep disturbance questionnaires were completed by caregivers of demented participants, whereas non-demented participants in the control group completed the questionnaire themselves (22)."
2	Page 32, lines 11 and 16: "cognitive screening instruments" - Define "screening" as used here. To me, screening means evaluation of asymptomatic individuals; you may not mean that here. Or reword, e.g. "which brief mental status instruments were used..."	We have reworded the phrase as suggested.

Reviewer	Comment	Response
3	My concern is that the literature is misrepresented. I do not think some of these papers can be correctly interpreted in the way you are trying to do here (particularly the behavioral signs and sleep sections). For the performance of the screening tests themselves, strong bias is exerted in the way the studies were done. To ignore these methodological issues is to present data that is much skewed from the actual performance of these instruments in a primary care setting.	Noted - specific responses detailed below.
3	This is a difficult literature. Results from the VA primary care population that would be most directly relevant aren't available because of the time it has taken us to get things written up. Still, I think you need to at least factor in the likely bias introduced by the published papers. I have detailed comments below. The performance of these tests is very different than that you present, supporting the idea that bias was introduced in the study design.	Noted - specific responses detailed below. Also, we had completed extensive quality evals of studies and will include these in our appendices.
3	I wouldn't put too much emphasis on that one meta analysis (ref 15). The individual studies included in the cross sectional analyses had some pretty iffy ways that dementia was called. For instance, the mmse is so insensitive that by the time a patient has crossed their threshold, the impairment was too far advanced for subjective memory complaints to be relevant to a case finding scenario in the clinic. I would have similar concerns about the use of a telephone screener to establish a diagnosis of dementia.	We re-wrote this section and tried to highlight more the deficiencies of some of the included studies.
3	I think the use of ADAS-Cog for diagnosis of dementia is questionable also. There may be some who would support it, but it is hardly a 'gold standard' as you call it (ref 35).	Noted and manuscript updated
3	Ref 36 had a good cognitive evaluation but this study examined different definitions of mci. When one of the criteria for diagnosis is subjective memory complaints, it does not seem valid to then look at how subjective memory complaints do as an indicator of the diagnosis.	Noted in manuscript
3	Ref 37 used an informant interview as their 'gold standard'. This was done with 121 subjects who screened positive and 35 who screened negative on a brief screen. While I believe that informant information is more valuable in this area that patient subjective memory complaint, I don't think this is a valid diagnostic method. This study establishes the level of correlation between patient complaint and informant complaint, nothing more.	Noted in manuscript

Reviewer	Comment	Response
3	As for reference 40, again the telephone screener was the primary means of evaluation. I suspect many, many milder cases were missed. Additionally, the subjective memory complaint was based solely on the question "do you have severe memory impairment?" as reported on a mailed questionnaire. I don't know of validation of this method, and it isn't really a straightforward inquiry into subjective memory problems. You go on to say that this method could classify healthy individuals as demented thus exaggerating reported specificity. The risk is actually higher the other way, I'd posit.	Noted and this study was de-emphasized
3	How did ref 43 get included? It doesn't compare prevalence rates of subjective memory impairment in those with and without dementia.	True - it compares SMC in patients with various levels of cognitive performance, but does not establish dementia diagnoses -- will exclude
3	Starting on line 15 of page 14 under the heading "Detailed Description" the use of MMSE is incorrect here. The Cache County study used an expanded and considerably more sensitive modified mini mental state exam or 3MS. I also believe you are misrepresenting/misunderstanding this study. While 61% of the demented subjects had behavioral disturbances in the past month (hardly low symptom prevalence as you state), this study documented behavioral problems in dementia and was not intended to address the use of behavioral symptoms in screening.	Thanks for clarifying - we will amend the report accordingly re: the modified MMSE. We hadn't intended to represent this as a study of use of behavioral sx for screening. Rather, the study was intended to test the hypothesis that in a community-based sample, demented patients would have more neuropsychiatric sx than non-demented patients. This may be useful for case-finding - ie - which sx should prompt a primary care physician to assess for dementia. Many clinicians may not think to assess one for dementia if presenting with sx such as apathy. Re: sx prevalence, we had meant to say neuropsych sx were common, but the prevalence of any one sx was relatively low. We will clarify in the report.
3	Page 15, line 17/18, do you mean the accuracy of dementia documentation in medical records of persons with and without dementia or with and without depression? If it is the former there is a whole literature that you ignore that concerns the documentation of a dementia diagnosis in the primary care setting.	We meant the latter - we do reference the former issue in the background section.
3	For reference 20, given that the average mmse of those they consider undiagnosed dementia was 17, I suspect they missed the mild cases. A MMSE of 17 isn't on the borderline of diagnosis. I'm also not convinced of their depression diagnoses, but setting aside the inadequacies of the diagnoses, I wouldn't jump to the conclusion that "some persons with mild dementia may have been misclassified as being depressed" (page 15, line 22/23). I don't think they caught those with mild dementia but the relationship between depression and dementia is nuanced and complex for even experienced geriatricians and geriatric psychiatrists.	Agreed - last statement was cut.

Reviewer	Comment	Response
3	You cannot look at a sample of Parkinson's disease patients and say anything about sleep and dementia except in the specific case of sleep and dementia in Parkinson's disease (top page 16).	We agree - our statement is meant to refer only to this study, but we will make clearer in the text that the results don't apply to patients with other types of dementia.
3	Reference 21 is incomplete.	It had originally been published online - we fixed the ref
3	Reference 28 is too old for me to access it electronically, but if frontal release signs were present in over half the participants, this is a severely demented group of subjects and not relevant to your topic.	Mean MMSE scores in the demented group were about 21 and suggested this was not a group with severe dementia. I agree this was not representative of a screen-diagnosed group of patients, but the findings may be relevant to case-finding discussions. Also interesting is that 9% of controls had release signs.
3	Reference 27 is also available to me only in abstract, but the abstract says 'with the exceptions of impaired vibration sense, loss of upward gaze, and bradykinesia, all signs were associated with the neurodegenerative syndromes and stroke' which seems different than what you report.	The abstract is slightly misleading - many of the signs were associated with stroke and/or Parkinsons, not dementia. The signs we mentioned were the ones associated with dementia. The study has numerous flaws in any case.
3	Reference 30 correlates an individual's assessment of their driving ability with that of an experienced neurologist and a driving instructor. It doesn't address use of driving skills as a screen for cognitive ability. Again, I think you misrepresent the literature.	It technically fit our inclusion criteria - I agree it's not a very useful study and we amended the paragraph to clarify the focus of the paper (was in the table, but I agree could have been clearer).
3	For reference 48, can you really report sensitivities of the Short Blessed (BOMC) of 100%? The 'field diagnoses' of dementia are suspect. Those felt to be demented were invited to Duke for a real evaluation. There were seven of these. The Short Blessed is brief and easily memorized by clinicians and requires no props. It is not, however, a test with a sensitivity of 100%.	We agree that sensitivity may be overestimated because 13 of subjects had a documented history of dementia, among the 26 identified as probably demented by field diagnosis. We have noted this limitation in Table 4 and in the text of the Results, in the BOMC section. Because the field methods used DSM criteria as a guide, the study meets our criteria for inclusion. However, we have replaced the results from this study in Table 5 with the results from Stuss 1996, a memory clinic sample that did not include patients who had been previously diagnosed with dementia.
3	Ref 49, again too old to pull up, seems to focus on severe dementia. Do your reported sens/spec come from a severely demented subgroup?	The sample in this study (Stuss 1996) consisted of patients who had been referred to a memory clinic for possible dementia, including some who on successive evaluations turned out not to have dementia. The final diagnosis was determined subsequent to the BOMC test. Although the results of the referral sample may not be applicable to primary care populations, the patients did not have a history of dementia. It does not appear that the sens/spec results were weighted by a more severely demented subgroup.

Reviewer	Comment	Response
3	Why is there a paragraph on informant reports of memory loss on pg 28? Again, you ignore a whole literature on this topic to focus on this paper?	We agree that this paragraph was not relevant to this section, and have removed it accordingly.
3	I really think that you ought to stress more that the six measures you look at are chosen by an 'expert panel' for various clinical reasons, not for rigorous scientific reasons. This was a series of phone conferences with people who were tasked with finding alternatives to the MMSE.	We agree, and have added text to the Methods section to indicate that the six measures reviewed were based on several clinical criteria.
3	The mini-Cog was not actually administered in MoVIES (ref 56) or in the University of Washington ADC (ref 64). Items incorporated in testing actually done were pulled to create a miniCog score. In actual practice, the sensitivities of the miniCog are considerably lower. Again, a brief test, easily remembered by clinicians and requiring no props except a paper and pencil, but not that sensitive.	We have added text to the Results to clarify that the Mini-Cog results from these studies were derived from components of longer tests, and that these results may not be directly comparable to the use of the Mini-Cog by itself in practice.
3	The diagnosis of dementia in ref 54 was based purely on informant interview, no cognitive testing. Not sufficient. Also, half of this ADC population was made up of non English speakers. How many of the informants spoke sufficient English to give a good history?	The study notes that non-English speakers were administered cognitive tests by foreign-born native speakers who were also fluent in English, although it is not explicitly specified that non-English speaking informants were interviewed likewise by an interpreter. However, we agree that this study does not meet criteria for the use of a full reference standard such as DSM-IV, because diagnostic workup for dementia was based on positive informant history, regardless of other patient evaluations that were conducted. We thank you for bringing this to our attention. We have excluded this study from our review.
3	It doesn't appear that investigators actually did any cognitive testing to arrive at a dementia diagnosis for the SLUMS study (ref 61). You comment on the inclusion of MCI in their population. They did not diagnose MCI (and could not without some testing) but rather a "mild neurocognitive disorder." There isn't such a diagnosis in DSM IV that I know of.	In Tariq 2006, the Methods state that each participant was evaluated during a routine clinic visit, a history was obtained from corroborating sources, a complete physical and mental status exam was performed, and lab findings were reviewed. Based on these data (which included a mental status exam) the investigators appear to have used, and state that they used, DSM-IV criteria to diagnose dementia. We concur that MCI is not a DSM-IV diagnosis; individuals with MCI fit neither criteria for normal or demented. Because different studies dealt differently with this subgroup, and some excluded them from analyses altogether, we noted how their inclusion could affect results.

Reviewer	Comment	Response
3	Page 32 under the heading of "Qualitative studies of the GPCOG and the Mini-Cog". This is a purely volunteer sample of clinicians. For a questionnaire with a 25% response rate (less actually since that 25% seems to be those who completed any part of the survey and there were the most responses familiar with the MMSE), there were 88% of respondents unfamiliar with the GPCOG and 75% unfamiliar with the Mini-Cog. This suggests giving weight to the 35 practitioners who said they had heard of the GPCOG and the 73 who said they'd heard of the miniCog.	We agree, and have removed the qualitative studies. We contacted the author of the IPA survey, who clarified that respondents rated the perceived quality on those tests with which they had some familiarity. Consequently the results for the GPCOG and Mini-Cog are based on a small, potentially biased sample. The 2nd qualitative study examined 2 of the 6 VA measures and ranked them equally high. Therefore we have noted in Future Research Recommendations that similar surveys be conducted among VA providers for input on the use of the 6 measures in practice.
3	As for the acceptability of screening, please note that you are basing your section primarily on one investigator using samples very different from the VA where we have had much better response from the Veterans concerning cognitive screening.	We have made note in the Results for KQ3 that 2 of the 3 studies were led by the same investigator. We have also removed some of the details about the studies and kept the more general findings, because these studies do not provide direct evidence about the 6 cognitive measures used in VA.
5	I found this report very informative overall and it does justice to this large body of literature pertaining to this important topic.	Noted.

APPENDIX E. GLOSSARY

<u>Agnosia</u>: Failure to recognize or identify objects despite intact sensory function.

<u>Alzheimer's disease (AD)</u>: A disease usually characterized by loss of memory, especially for learning new information, reflecting deterioration in the functioning of the medial temporal lobe and hippocampus areas of the brain. Later in the illness, other higher functions of the cerebral cortex become affected: these include language, praxis (putting theoretical knowledge into practice) and executive function (involved in processes such as planning, abstract thinking, rule acquisition, initiating appropriate actions and inhibiting inappropriate actions, and selecting relevant sensory information). Behavioral and psychiatric disturbances are also seen, which include depression, apathy, agitation, disinhibition, psychosis (delusions and hallucinations), wandering, aggression, incontinence and altered eating habits.

<u>Aphasia</u>: Deterioration in language skills, such as word-finding difficulties, reduction in output, loss of fluency, and poor comprehension.

<u>Apraxia</u>: Total or partial loss of the ability to perform coordinated movements or manipulate objects in the absence of motor or sensory impairment.

<u>Case-finding</u>: The strategy of identifying a new occurrence of disease among patients selected on the presence of risk factors, signs, or symptoms.

<u>Cohort</u>: A group of persons with a common characteristic or set of characteristics. Typically, the group is followed for a specified period of time to determine the incidence of a disorder or complication of an established disorder (prognosis).

<u>Cohort Study: (Cohort Analytic Study)</u>: Prospective investigation of the factors that might cause a disorder in which a cohort of individuals who do not have evidence of an outcome of interest but who are exposed to the putative cause are compared with a concurrent cohort who are also free of the outcome but not exposed to the putative cause. Both cohorts are then followed to compare the incidence of the outcome of interest. Used for Prospective Study.

<u>Dementia</u>: The development of multiple cognitive deficits that include memory impairment and at least 1 of the following cognitive disturbances: agnosia, aphasia, apraxia, or a disturbance in executive functioning. Deficits must be severe enough to cause significant decline in social or occupational functioning and must represent a decline from previous baseline functioning.

<u>Dementia with Lewy bodies (DLB)</u>: One of the most common types of progressive dementia and shares characteristics with both Alzheimer's and Parkinson's diseases. Its central feature is progressive cognitive decline, combined with three additional defining features: pronounced fluctuations in alertness and attention, such as frequent drowsiness, lethargy, lengthy periods of time spent staring into space or disorganised speech; recurrent visual hallucinations; and parkinsonian motor symptoms, such as rigidity and the loss of spontaneous movement. The symptoms of DLB are caused by the build-up of Lewy bodies (protein deposits found in nerve cells) in areas of the brain that control particular aspects of memory and motor control.

<u>Executive Functioning</u>: The ability to think abstractly and to plan, initiate, sequence, monitor, and stop complex behavior.

Graphesthesia: The ability to recognize a number or letter written on the skin by the sensation of touch.

Heterogeneity: A term used to illustrate the variability or differences between studies in the estimates of effects.

Incidence: The number of new cases of a disease per population over a given time period. Incidence measures how frequently a new case of disease occurs, as opposed to prevalence, which conveys how widespread a disease is in a population.

Inter-rater reliability: A measure of the extent to which multiple raters or judges agree when providing a rating, scoring, or assessment.

Key questions: Questions posed by the advisory panel that are used to guide the identification and interrogation of the evidence base relevant to the topic of the guideline.

Likelihood Ratio: For a screening or diagnostic test (including clinical signs or symptoms), expresses the relative likelihood that a given test result would be expected in a participant with (as opposed to one without) a disorder of interest.

Mild Cognitive Impairment (MCI): Presence of a memory complaint, preferably corroborated by an informant, objective memory impairment, and normal general cognitive function. Activities of daily living are intact and the patient does not meet clinical criteria for dementia.

Neuropsychiatric symptoms: Symptoms which generally fall within one of three symptom clusters: agitation, psychosis and mood disorders. Symptoms of agitation often include aggressiveness or irritability. Symptoms of psychosis are hallucinations – auditory or visual, and delusions. Mood disorders would include depression and anxiety.

Odds ratio: A ratio of the odds of having the disease of interest in a group with a particular exposure, symptom, or characteristic of interest, to the odds of disease in a group that does not have the exposure /symptom / characteristic. An odds ratio of 1 indicates that the disease is equally likely to occur in both groups. On odds ratio of 4 indicates that the disease is 4 times more likely to be present in the group that has the symptom or characteristic of interest, compared with the group that does not have this symptom.

Predictive Value (PPV): Positive Predictive Value – the proportion of people with a positive test who have the disease; Negative Predictive Value – proportion of people with a negative test who are free of disease.

Prevalence: The total number of cases of the disease in the population at a given time, expressed as a proportion in which the number of cases is the numerator and the population at risk is the denominator.

Release signs: Primitive reflexes that are normally present in infants, including the suck, snout, palmomental, and grasp reflexes. They are seen in disorders that affect the frontal lobes, such as dementias, metabolic encephalopathies, closed head trauma, and hydrocephalus.

Remote/over-learned memory: The ability to remember people or events from the distant past, or over-learned information such as the days in the week or one's birthday.

Registration/recall: The processing of received information, and the retrieval of the information in response to a cue for use in a process or activity.

Screening: A strategy used in a population to detect a disease in individuals without signs or symptoms of that disease. Universal screening involves screening of all individuals in a certain category, for example, all persons age 65 and older.

Screening test: A brief instrument used to determine the likelihood of whether a disease may be present, and whether more comprehensive diagnostic testing may be needed. The predictive value of a screening test is influenced by the prevalence of the disease in the population. In universal screening, a screening test would be administered to all persons in a certain category (e.g. age 65+). In a case-finding approach, the screening test would be selectively administered when a patient has risk factors or presents with signs or symptoms of the disease.

Sensitivity: The proportion of people who truly have a designated disorder who are so identified by the test. The test may consist of, or include, clinical observations. The proportion of truly diseased persons in the screened population who are identified as diseased by the screening test—that is, the true-positive rate.

Specificity: The proportion of people who are truly free of a designated disorder who are so identified by the test. The test may consist of, or include, clinical observations. The proportion of truly nondiseased persons who are identified as such by the screening test—that is, the true-negative rate.

Stereognosis: The ability to perceive the form of an object by using the sense of touch.

Sources

American Psychiatric Association. *Diagnostic and Statistical Manual of Mental Disorders*, Fourth Edition, Text Revision. Washington, DC: American Psychiatric Association, 2000.

Guyatt G, Rennie D. User's Guides to the Medical Literature: A manual for evidence-based clinical practice. Chicago: AMA Press, 2002.

Holsinger T, Deveau J, Boustani M, Williams JW, Jr. Does this patient have dementia? JAMA 2007;297(21):2391-404.

National Institute for Health and Clinical Excellence (NICE). Dementia: A NICE–SCIE Guideline on supporting people with dementia and their carers in health and social care. In: National Clinical Practice Guideline Number 42: The British Psychological Society and Gaskell; 2007.

Petersen RC, Stevens JC, Ganguli M, Tangalos EG, Cummings JL, DeKosky ST. Practice parameter: early detection of dementia: mild cognitive impairment (an evidence-based review). Report of the Quality Standards Subcommittee of the American Academy of Neurology. Neurology 2001;56(9):1133-42.

Walker, HK. The suck, snout, palmomental, and grasp reflexes. *Clinical Methods – the History, Physical, and Laboratory Examinations*. Third Edition. Butterworth Publishers, 1990.

West S, King V, Carey TS, et al. Systems to rate the strength of scientific evidence: Evidence Report/Technology Assessment, Number 47. Rockville, MD: Agency for Healthcare Research and Quality. AHRQ Publication No. 02-E016, April 2002.

www.ingramcontent.com/pod-product-compliance
Lightning Source LLC
Chambersburg PA
CBHW081613170526
45166CB00009B/2951